INSTANT HEALTH: THE SHAOLIN

QIGONG

WORKOUT FOR LONGEVITY

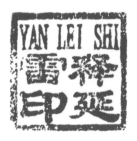

SHIFU YAN LEI

YAN LEI

Published by Yan Lei Press
www.shifuyanlei.co.uk
Text copyright © Yan Lei
Photographic copyright © Manuel Vason

First Published November 2009

Photos taken on location at the Huangshan mountain,
the Shaolin Temple, and Shaolin Village China.

ISBN: 978-0-9563101-0-1
A catalogue record for this book is available from
the British Library.
Printed and bound in China.

CREDITS
Photography: Manuel Vason, ManuelVason@MVStudio,
www.mvstudio.net
Book design: Andrew Egan and Amy Gustantino, CoolGraySeven,
www.CoolGraySeven.com
Editor: Cat Goscovitch
Martial Arts technical advisor: ShifuYang Hong Zhou,
www.yhzsz.com

DISCLAIMER
THE WORKOUT PROGRAM IN THIS BOOK MAY
NOT BE APPROPRIATE FOR EVERYONE. AS WITH
ALL EXERCISE PROGRAMS, YOU SHOULD GET
YOUR DOCTOR'S APPROVAL BEFORE BEGINNING.
THE AUTHOR AND PUBLISHER IS NOT RESPONSIBLE
NOR LIABLE FOR ANY HARM OR INJURY RESULTING
FROM THIS PROGRAM.

Thank you to my master the Shaolin Abbot; Shi Yong Xin for giving me the opportunity to train at the Shaolin Temple, and giving me a strong mind and willpower. Big thank you to my blood and kung fu brother Shifu Yan Zi. You are not just my brother, you are also in some ways my martial art's teacher. Without your experience I could not have done this book. Thank you to my family for giving me a lot of positive energy.

Thank you to Cat Goscovitch for researching, editing, and producing this book. Manuel Vason for having the energy to follow me round China, climb mountains, get bitten by mosquitoes in bamboo forests, suffer from food poisoning, and still manage to take such stunning photographs. And also Alex Tovey for assisting him and us on the China trip, and shooting the documentary footage.

Thank you to my kung fu brother Shifu Yang Hong Zhou for his technical advice and hospitality at his school. Thank you to Andrew Egan and Amy Gustantino at CoolGraySeven for designing such a beautiful book. And my first readers Anna Owen and Dr Janusz Piotrowicz for your valuable feedback.

I'm very fortunate to have a fantastic team who work tirelessly on my behalf to help promote authentic Shaolin. I couldn't do it without them. My DVD director and editor Marek Budzynski. Thank you to Marcus Taylor at www.taylorthomas.co.uk for designing my website and DVD's.

Thank you to all of my loyal students for your support and trust.

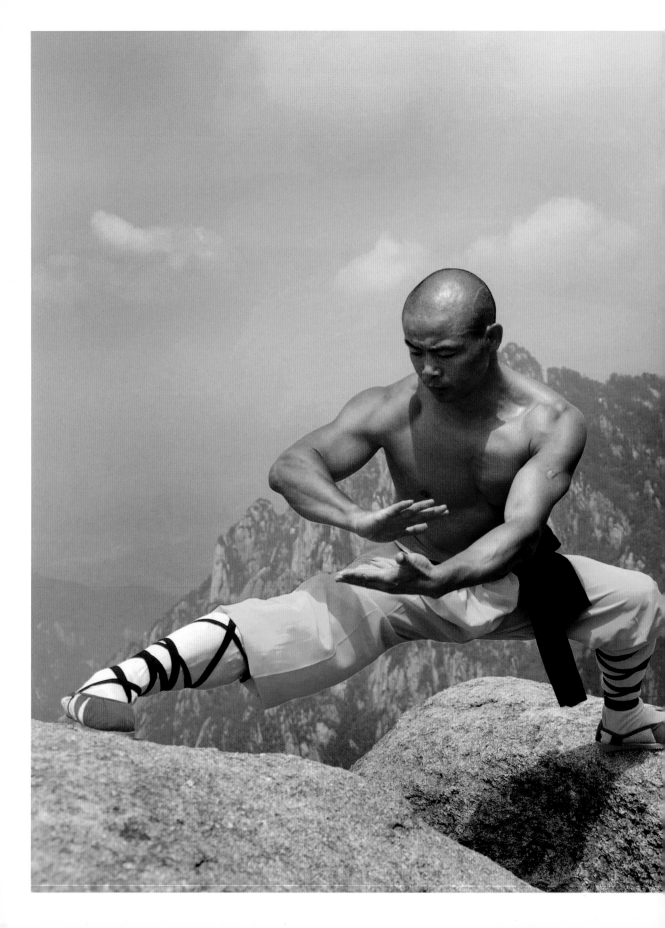

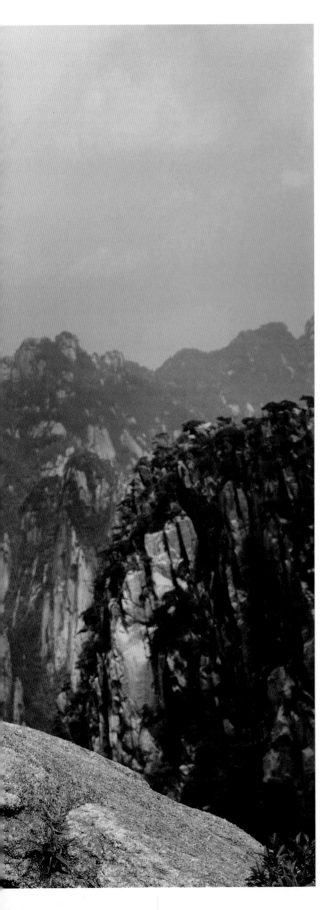

"ALTHOUGH LIFE-EXPECTANCY HAS INCREASED, IT HAS NOT DONE SO AT THE SAME RATE AS 'HEALTHY' LIFE-EXPECTANCY, MEANING THAT PEOPLE ARE NOW SPENDING MORE YEARS IN POOR HEALTH."

Mintel – Healthy Lifestyle Report 2008

PREFACE

Most of us agree that good health is not just about being free of illness or disease. We want peace of mind and high levels of energy so we can enjoy our life, but many of us tend to work all day at a computer and this can leave us feeling drained. A recent study by Dr Nakazawa from Chiba University in Japan concluded that regular computer use was responsible for headaches, joint pain, insomnia and fatigue.

To get us through the day many of us use caffeine and sugar, which has a yoyo effect on our blood sugar level and puts a strain on our hormonal system and can lead to an increase in stress and anxiety. In a study in 2003 by Shedon Cohen, stress was seen to depress the immune system.

As we get older our unhealthy lifestyle may lead to illnesses such as diabetes, high cholesterol, high blood pressure and joint problems. An increase in cardiovascular disease has resulted in large part from our unhealthy lifestyle and increased number of working hours. Modern medicine means that we can live longer but our standard of living is not what it should be.

Exercise helps to reduce some of these health problems but many of us simply don't have the energy to do it, and rather than being something pleasurable, it can feel like a chore.

For those of us who are engaged in an exercise programme, even though we are increasingly aware of the mind-body connection, we still tend to separate the mind and body out. We go to the gym for a workout and a yoga class for flexibility. To de-stress our mind we go on holiday or have a massage. Both types of lifestyle are out of balance and do not address the major issues that threaten our health and energy levels.

Fifteen hundred years ago, Buddhist monks at the Shaolin Temple in China suffered from many of the same problems we face today. In their quest for enlightenment they sat for long hours, and as a result, their bodies became weak and their minds dull. Not having access to caffeine or sugar they had to find other ways to boost their health and energy.

An Indian monk called Bodhidharma created special breathing exercises called Qigong. These methods were shown to be effective not only at increasing their energy but prolonging life. The monks then combined Qigong with Kung Fu to increase their martial power and this is what the Shaolin Temple has become famous for today.

You may have seen Shaolin Monks demonstrate their "super human" skills on stage and screen. These are not lofty techniques reserved exclusively for Shaolin monks but exercises that are accessible to all. Time-tested for thousands of years, latest research shows that these ancient movements are a powerful longevity tool that can protect us against a wide range of health problems including insomnia, poor digestion, high blood pressure, backache, and computer-related stress. Modern science is discovering that the mind and body are not separate from each other but interdependent, and a mind at peace with itself protects the body's health.

That principle is fundamental at the Shaolin Temple. We believe that health and fitness is not just about aerobic activity and eating well, we also need to have strong internal organs and mental and spiritual balance. The key to achieving this is through a finely tuned balance of Qigong and Kung Fu or another exercise that includes cardiovascular and strength training. When we are young we practise more Kung Fu than Qigong and as we get older we practise more Qigong than Kung Fu.

This method of training means that Shaolin exercises can be adapted to suit any life stage: teen years, middle and advanced years. Some of the Qigong exercises can even be done in just a few minutes a day so we can easily fit them into our hectic lifestyle.

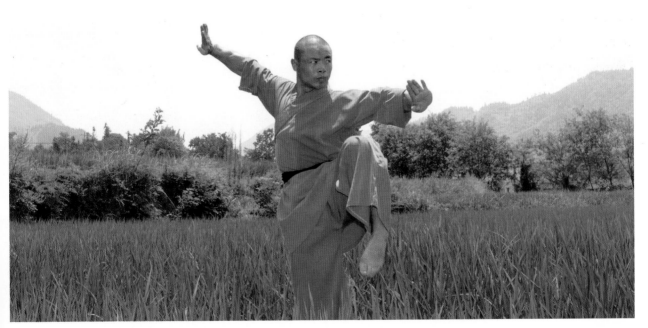

The teachings that appear in this book were originally passed down secretly from generation to generation at the Shaolin Temple in China. Bodhidharma was the 1st generation and I am one of the 34th generation. In 1985 the Chinese government granted its approval of Qigong and I have been given permission to teach what I learnt at the Temple.

For those of you who are investigating Shaolin for the first time, this book offers a clear path so you can quickly get to the heart of the practice. For people already familiar with Shaolin, including long-term practitioners, this book provides a long-needed authentic guide to the essential exercises we perform at the Shaolin Temple, free of the secrets and myths that have accumulated in the West.

Shaolin is not just a form of exercise but an art like music or literature, which enables us to understand our lives and find peace within ourselves. At the Shaolin Temple we believe it is best to prevent disease rather than curing it when it occurs. In this book I give you precise instructions as to how you can achieve this.

Amituofo,

Shifu Shi Yan Lei

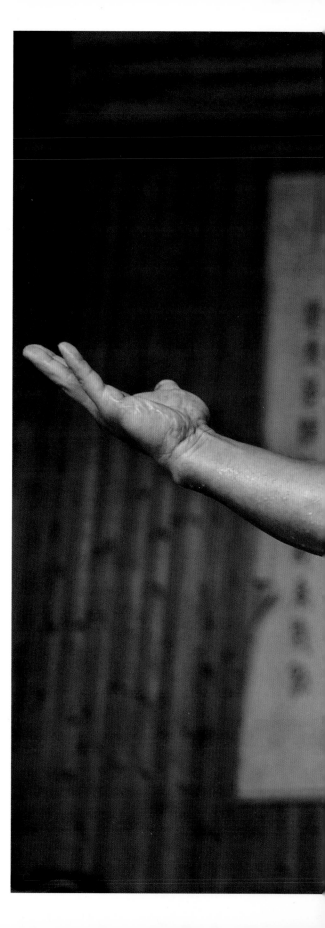

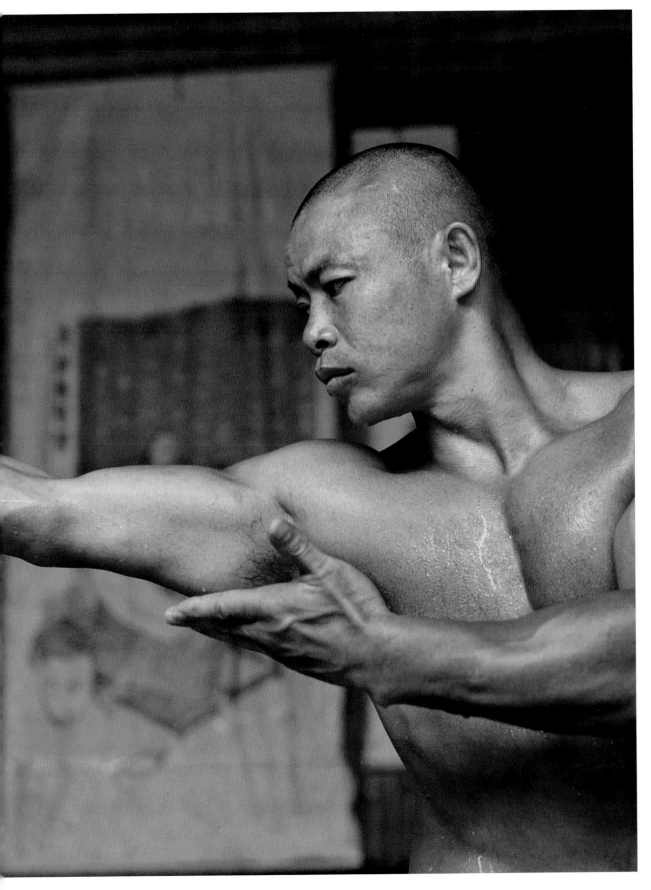

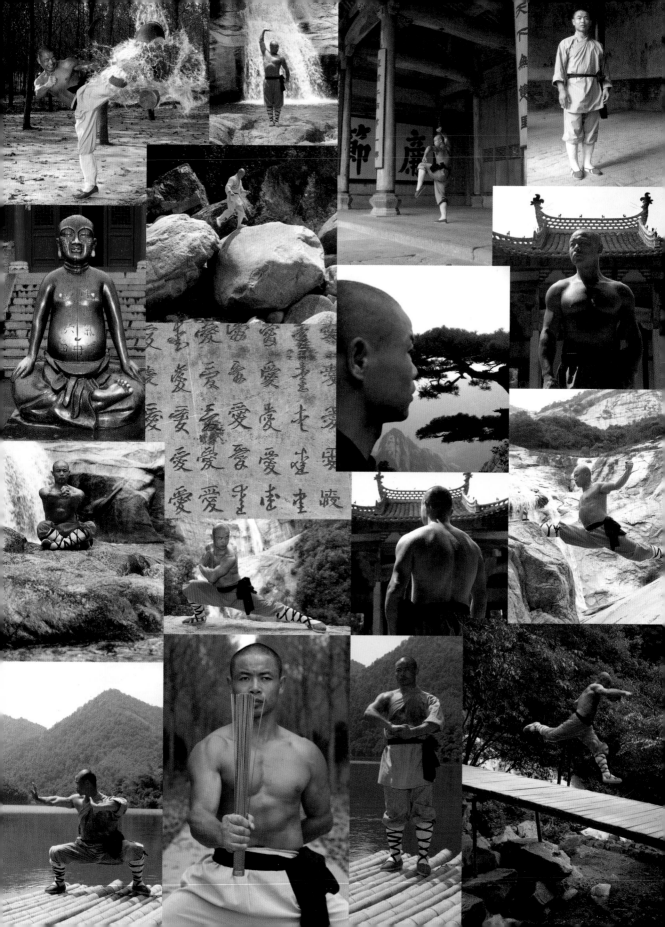

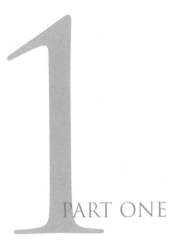

PART ONE

THE ART AND SCIENCE OF SHAOLIN TEMPLE LONGEVITY

PART TWO

2

THE FUNDAMENTALS OF SHAOLIN QIGONG

PART THREE

3

THE QIGONG WORKOUT FOR LONGEVITY

PART ONE
THE ART AND SCIENCE OF SHAOLIN TEMPLE LONGEVITY

CHAPTER ONE

WHAT IS SHAOLIN QIGONG?

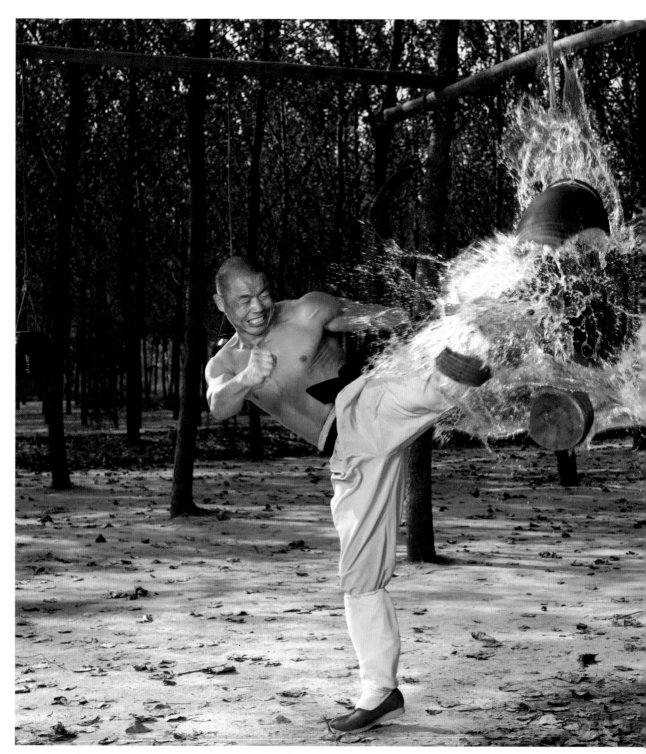

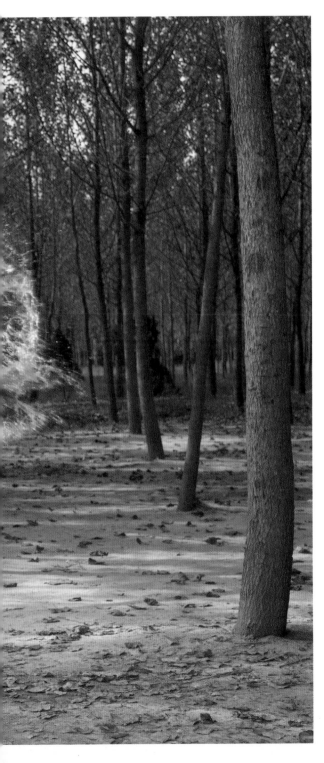

"ITS TRAINING
HAS ITS ORDER,
ITS METHODS
INCLUDE
INTERNAL AND
EXTERNAL.
QI MUST BE
TRANSPORTED
AND USED,
MOVING HAS
BEGINNING
AND STOPPING."

If aerobic exercise were the key to great health, then top athletes, footballers and boxers would be the healthiest people in the world, yet most of them retire when they are still young. They tend to suffer from injuries and have an array of physiotherapists and sport's masseurs to keep their body on top form. This is because they only look after the exterior of their body, the parts of the body which will serve them in their sport. They understand the importance of nutrition but they haven't yet understood the importance of Qi.

At the Shaolin Temple we put our bodies through the same rigorous exercise as an Olympian athlete yet we don't suffer the same level of illness or injury. Our monks never retire. On the contrary their training deepens as they get older.

SHARPENING THE KNIFE

At the Shaolin Temple we believe there are two actions we need to take for good health: use and look after. We will be unsuccessful if we separate the two. We can't just use and not look after or look after and not use. Most of us have a mistaken belief that we have to conserve our energy but this is like trying to gain something with a closed hand. Only when we have opened our hand can we gain something. Only when we have used our energy can we fully replenish it.

Professional chefs regularly sharpen their knives. Through experience they know that it is worth taking the time to do this because it increases the knife's effectiveness and prolongs its life. It is the same with our bodies. We use our bodies through the practice of Kung Fu and we look after our bodies through the practice of Qigong.

SHAOLIN QIGONG (pronounced chee gong)

If a mobile phone gets low in energy then it beeps to let us know. Our bodies are the same. Our warning sign is when our thoughts start to circle or we feel under the weather, or we wake up in the morning still feeling tired. These are all signs that our Qi is running low. The regular practice of Qigong acts as a natural battery charger for the body and keeps our energy levels topped up.

No one word can capture the true meaning of Qi. It is sometimes translated as breath or vital energy but it is much more than this. We believe that a person contains a miniature Universe, and Qi is the inexhaustible energy of the Universe which underpins all of existence.

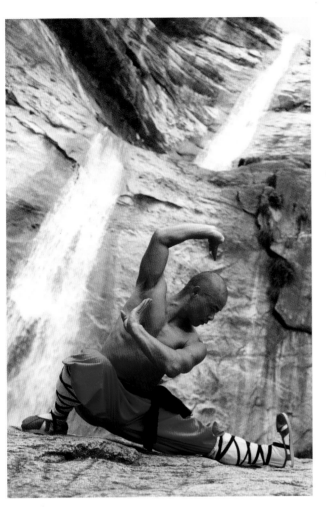

NO ONE WORD CAN CAPTURE THE TRUE MEANING OF QI.

IT IS SOMETIMES TRANSLATED AS BREATH OR VITAL ENERGY BUT IT IS MUCH MORE THAN THIS.

Gong means work and time. We put energy and time into working with our Qi to balance the Yin and the Yang, open the meridians and strengthen the internal organs. Qigong increases vitality because it conserves energy by lowering the metabolic rate. Through a series of breathing exercises, special movements and self-massage techniques we restore our body to its original programme of health. When these movements are linked together they are then called a "form".

KUNG FU

Kung Fu training consists of traditional forms that tap into the innate harmony and energy of our mind and body, strength-training techniques, and cardiovascular training. Kung Fu is not just for martial artists but for anyone who wants to achieve optimum fitness. Not only does Shaolin Kung Fu preserve muscle and bone mass as we grow older but it also increases our confidence as we discover that we have much greater abilities than we thought we had. If you already have a regular fitness programme then you don't need to learn kung fu, you can simply add in the Shaolin Qigong Workout from this book.

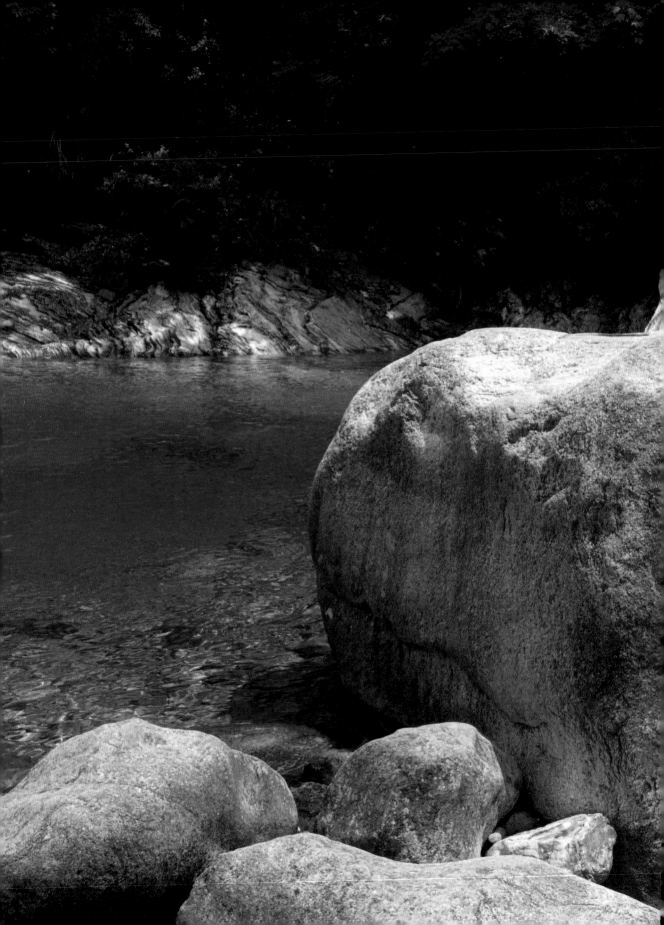

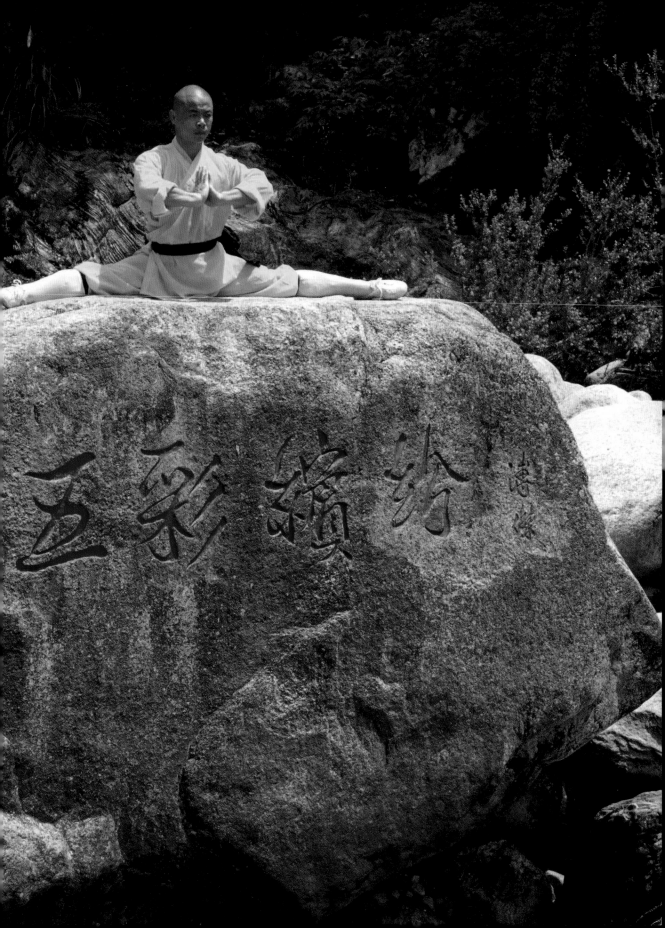

YIN AND YANG

Controlling the yang and yin elements by
embracing the one,
Can you not allow them to depart,
Concentrating the qi and
achieving utmost suppleness,
Can you not become like a child?

Dao De Jing

The character for Yin originally meant the shady side of the mountain and the character for Yang was the sunny side of the mountain. All things contain Yin and Yang. Night is Yin and day is Yang, earth is Yin and heaven is Yang, female is Yin and male is Yang, cold is Yin and heat is Yang, and so on. Yin and Yang are interdependent. Yin cannot exist without Yang and Yang cannot exist without Yin.

Within the body, inhaling is Yin and exhaling is Yang. Rest is Yin and activity is Yang. Yin and Yang are constantly changing and to balance these energies harmoniously we practise Qigong.

MERIDIANS

The Meridians move the Qi and blood,
regulate Yin and Yang,
moisten the tendons and bones,
benefit the joints.

Nei Jing Yang

Meridians are the energy matrix of our body. They are the invisible channels that link together all of our organs. They flow where the blood flows. When we are under stress the channels get blocked and this leads to physical and emotional illness. It is vital for our health that the Meridians are clear so that the Qi can flow properly.

MINDFULNESS

When you try to stop activity to achieve passivity,
Your very effort fills you with activity,
As long as you remain in one extreme or the other
You will never know Oneness.

Master Sengsban

Being present in the moment is called Mindfulness and it is one of the fundamental keys to banishing stress. Recent research from the Department of Psychology and Health at Tilburg University in the Netherlands found support for the effects of mindfulness as an individual stress reliever. It can also be used as an effective tool to help overcome depression.

When I trained at the Shaolin Temple, I was taught that every movement I did was a meditation; when I kicked I did kicking meditation and when I ran I did running meditation. My ordinary mind was already a Buddha mind and all of my training was enlightened activity. Training with this attitude helps us to let go of our problems and fully commit ourselves to the Shaolin Qigong Workout, so when we finish our training, we feel brand new.

If Buddha does not inspire you then you can substitute him for a Bodhisattva or God or the Tao. Use whatever helps you to let go of your small self and embrace the wisdom that surrounds you.

CHAPTER TWO

QIGONG: THE LONGEVITY MEDICINE

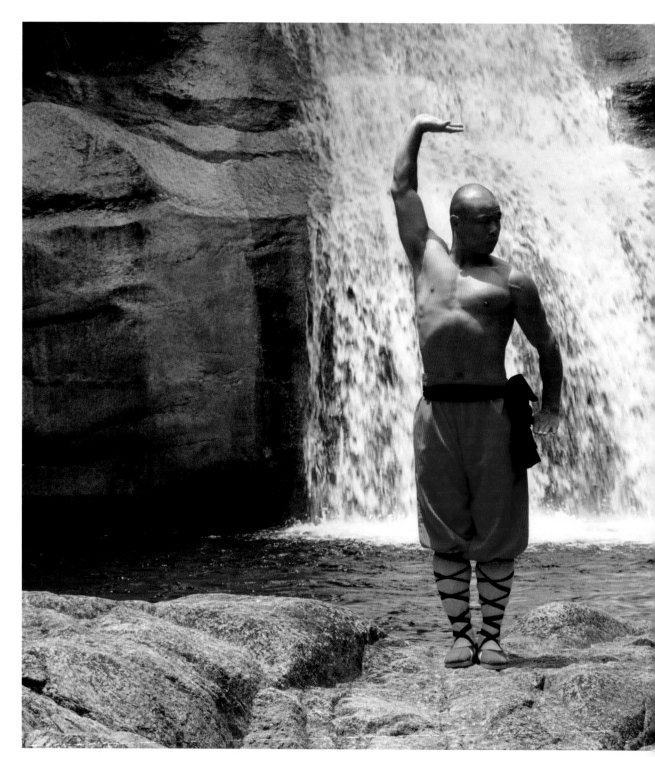

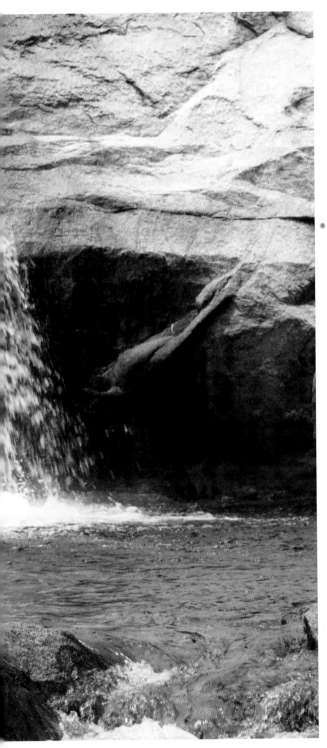

Good health, peace and contentment are our birthright. Many of the exercises at the Shaolin Temple were aimed at helping the monks realize enlightenment but today we can use these exercises for health and happiness in our everyday life. If we look after our body, this takes care of our mind and that in turn has a beneficial effect on our family and friends.

Each phase of our life offers unique challenges and the Shaolin Qigong Workout can help us in every decade. Its unique integration of stretching, Qigong, and self-massage gives us a direct path to optimum health. This workout coupled with a positive mental attitude, regular exercise, and a balanced diet can help us to live a longer and healthier life.

QIGONG AND EXERCISE

The exercises that I teach in this book are Qigong, but to balance our body we need to practise cardiovascular and strength training as well. If you already have an exercise regime that you are happy with, then all you have to do is add Qigong. If you're a jogger, then you can slot the Qigong form either before you start your run or after you've finished. If you are a member of a gym, then you can warm up or cool down with Qigong. Weight lifters will find it enhances their fitness programme, joggers will find that it gives them more energy and makes running easier. Yoga practioners will discover that Qigong complements and deepens their practice.

With yoga it's best to do the Qigong form at the end of your yoga practice, but with cardiovascular exercise it makes no difference whether you do it before or after. Experiment and find out which your body prefers.

For those of you who don't exercise, the Shaolin Qigong Workout can act as a gateway to build your mind and body to a level where exercise is possible. If you don't exercise because you find it a chore, then I recommend you learn Shaolin Kung Fu, as it's impossible to get bored with the rich array and variety of movements that it offers.

THE CRUCIAL PERCENTAGE FACTOR – OPTIMUM HEALTH AND FITNESS AT EVERY AGE

Some people train in Shaolin when they are six years old and others when they are sixty. Adapting Shaolin to suit these different ages is down to the crucial percentage factor of how much Qigong training and how much Kung Fu or exercise we do. At the Shaolin Temple we call Qigong internal training and Kung Fu external training.

A teenager will do about 95% external training and 5 % internal training. This means if he or she trains for one hour then the majority of his or her training will be Kung Fu. A sixty-year-old man or woman will do about 70% internal and 30 % external, depending on their fitness level. This means if they train for one hour, then they will do about 42 minutes of internal training and 18 minutes of external training. Or, if they train three times a week, then they may dedicate two of their training sessions to Qigong and one of their sessions to kung fu. As they get fitter or stronger this percentage may change.

There is no golden rule and our body is not a machine. Sometimes we feel stressed or tired and we don't have much energy to do any exercise so we do more internal training. The Shaolin Qigong Workout helps us to tune into our bodies so we instinctively know what we should do.

As a general rule, if you are older then you will do more Qigong training, but even if you are young, you should still look after your body through regular Qigong. This will help to prevent ageing and illness in the body before it happens.

MORE INTERNAL

"I'm tired after a day's work and don't want to do anything strenuous; I just want to relax."
"I regularly feel tired when I wake up in the morning."

If these statements apply to you, then I recommend that you start off by doing the Shaolin Qigong Workout. For those of you who feel drained of energy, you may find that after running through this sequence you will have an immediate increase in energy. If this is the case you can move on and do some exercise, or finish off with the Instant Health Massage.

"Exercise and diet aren't helping me to lose weight."

If you are exercising but not losing weight this maybe because your endocrine system is out of balance and your body may be producing too much cortisol. You need to balance it with a regular Qigong Workout.

"I haven't exercised since I was at school but my doctor has told me to start."

For those of you who are elderly or haven't exercised in a long time, then stick to the Qigong Workout and, when your body starts to feel fitter and more flexible, gently begin by adding some walking and then jogging in the park.

"Children should come with a health-warning! I've just had a baby and the last thing I want to do is exercise, I want some me time."

Qigong is a pleasurable activity that is something we can do to reduce stress and give something back to ourselves. A 2008 review of studies on mind-body interventions in pregnancy and childbirth found that it helped to reduce a mother's stress and anxiety.

"I'm starting to notice signs of ageing in my face and body."

In China, Qigong is called the secret of youth and longevity. In the past, Taoist and Buddhist monks wanted to live as long as possible so they could discover the secrets of life. Qigong enabled them to do this. The Qigong Workout coupled with The Instant Health Massage are great ways to slow down the ageing process.

MORE EXTERNAL

"I had a Shaolin session after a particularly bad day and it felt brilliant punching and kicking my frustration away."
"I already exercise but I'd like to find a technique to enhance what I do."
"I am a student who gets tired from sitting at college studying all day."
"I get stressed from running my own business and my time is limited so I need something that's going to give me a good cardiovascular workout."

Exercise is a stress-buster. Generally if you are under thirty and you are reasonably fit then you can do more external training than internal. Instead of starting with Qigong, you can end your session with Qigong to calm yourself down, regulate your Qi and bring it back to your body. Full details on external training can be found in my second book: *Instant Fitness: The Shaolin Kung Fu Workout.*

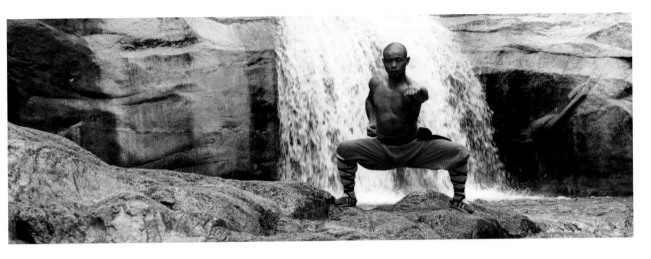

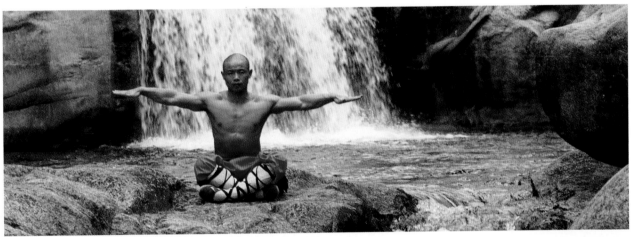

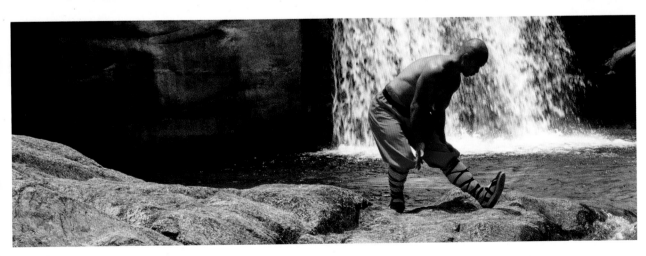

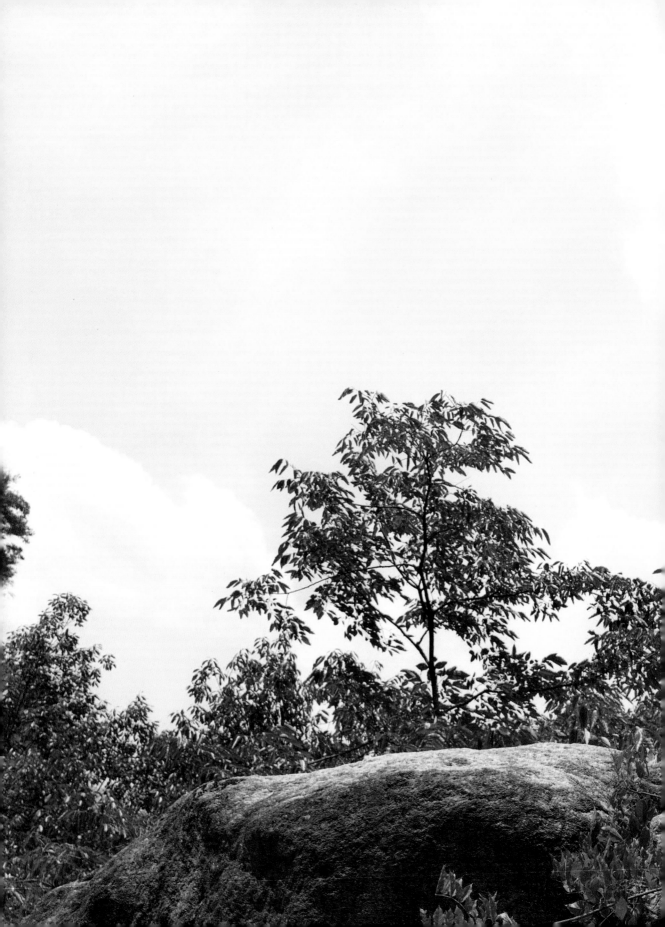

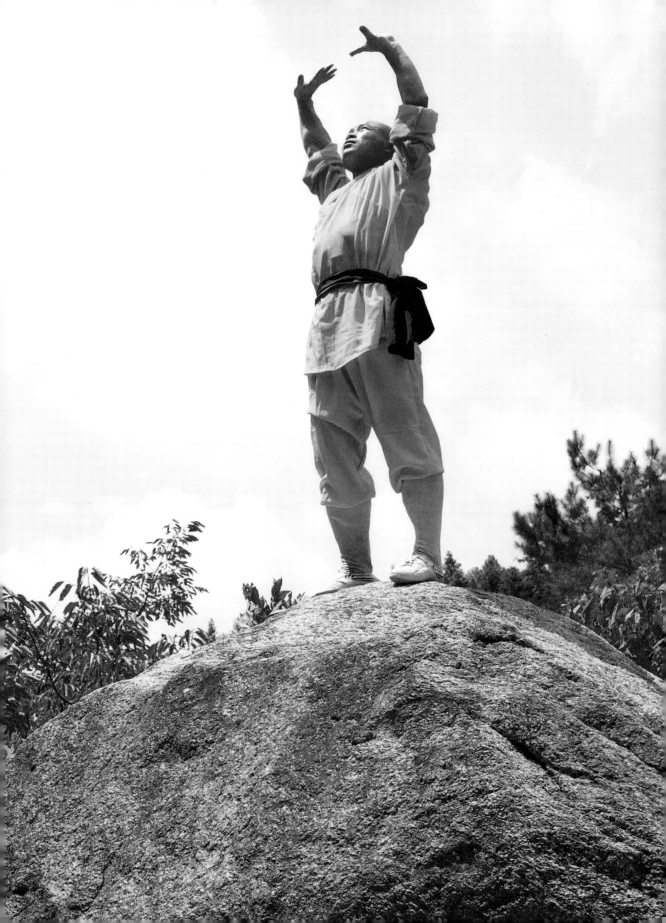

THE SHAOLIN QIGONG WORKOUT – A SUMMARY

The traditional Western way of maintaining health and fitness consists of eight steps:

Warm Up

Strength Training

Aerobic activity

Yoga for flexibility

Pilates to strengthen core muscles

Massage for relaxation

Meditation for mindfulness

Additional health supplements for energy and balance

The Instant Health Workout consists of four steps to wellness:

WARM UP
STRETCHING
QIGONG
SELF-MASSAGE

If you supplement this workout with a form of aerobic activity you are not only building your fitness but also your health. This is a project which is for your whole life so it is important that you are consistent and enjoy yourself. If you are not enjoying yourself then stop doing it and ask yourself, why not? Every body is different and the Shaolin Qigong Workout is a personalised workout that can help you to achieve your lifetime goal of health, fitness, and longevity.

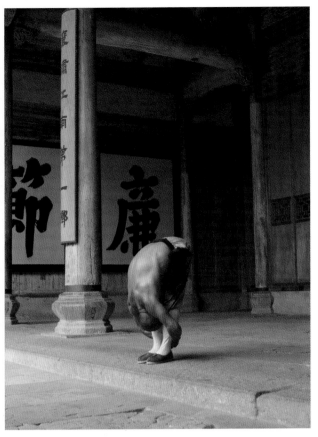
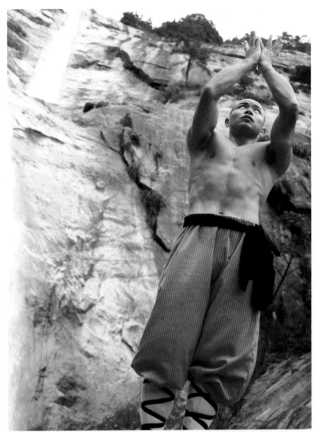
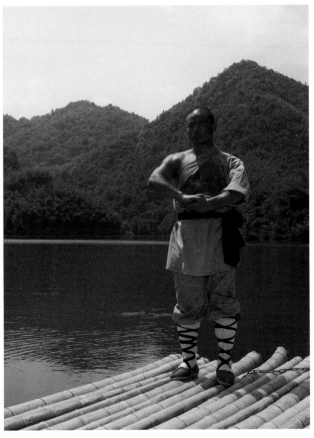
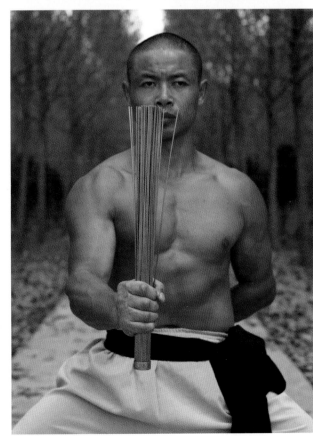

CHAPTER THREE

DOES QIGONG WORK? THE SCIENTIFIC EVIDENCE

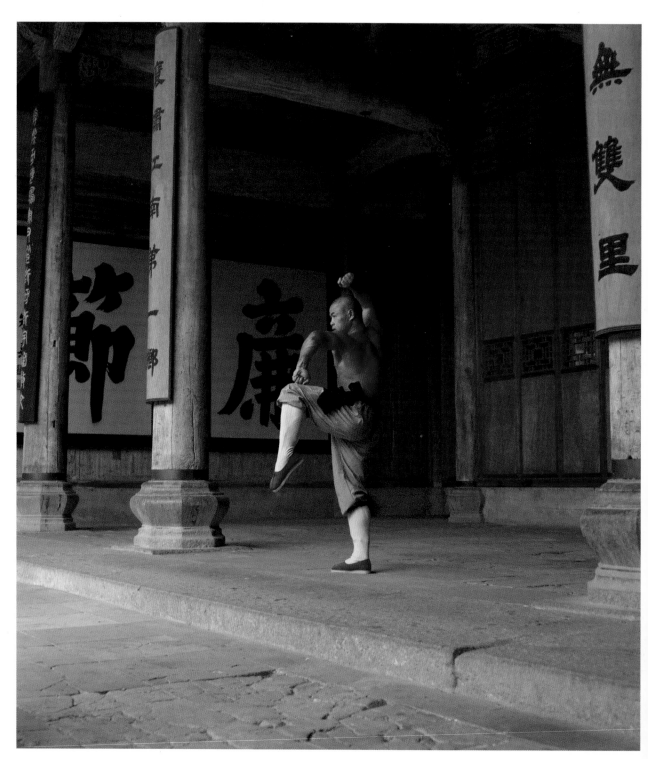

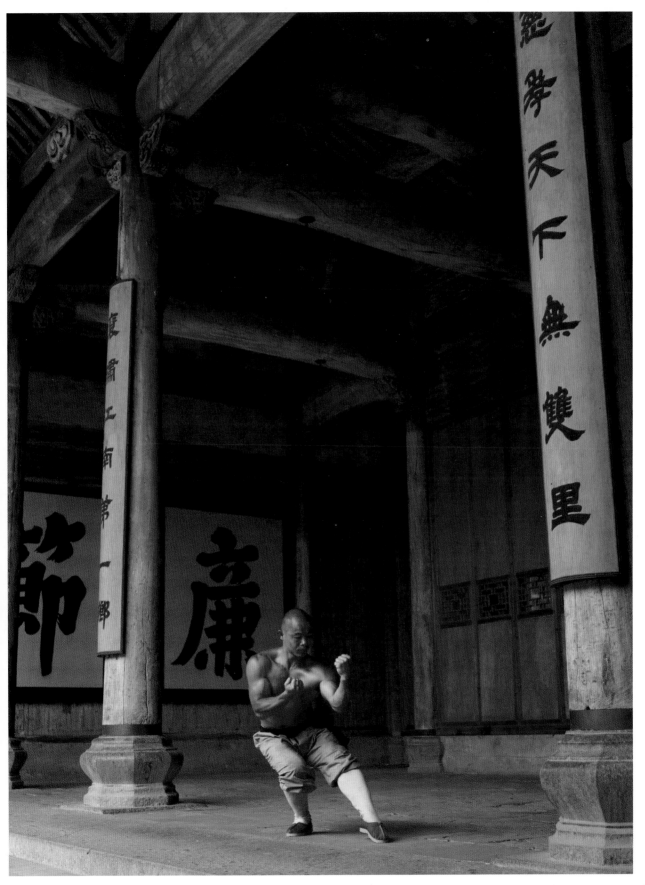

I have been teaching in the West for many years. Some of the changes my students have experienced are:

Improved mental clarity

Increase in energy levels

A deep feeling of peace

Relief from back pain

Increase in confidence

General feeling of wellness

They don't catch colds as often as before.

They don't suffer from headaches like they used to

A healthy glow to their skin

Weight loss

Regulation of blood pressure

Regulation of menstruation

It could be argued that some of these changes are a result of regular exercise. But I attribute the majority of these changes to the unique combination of exercise (external) and Qigong (internal). For more than fifteen hundred years Qigong has been used in the Shaolin Temple for martial power and health. Today, we can examine the results of experiments and clinical trials with Qigong practitioners.

QIGONG AND AGEING

It has been shown that practitioners of Qigong have higher levels of superoxide dismutase (SOD), an enzyme that protects cells against the build-up of the highly toxic free radical Superoxide, which can cause ageing - wrinkling and changes in skin pigmentation - in the same way that exposure to air causes food to perish. Superoxide can also cause the breakdown of cartilage and synovial fluid (the cushioning and lubrication between bones) leading to arthritis and joint damage, and has even been implicated as a causative agent in cancer and immune system disorder.

Research at Baylor Medical School in Texas has found that some cells from the bodies of long-term Qigong practitioners live five times longer than the same cells from ordinary test subjects.

Research from The Shanghai Institute of Hypertension looked at several aspects of ageing. They determined that Qigong is an effective measure in preventing and treating geriatric diseases and delaying the ageing process.

QIGONG AND COMPUTER RELATED STRESS INCLUDING BACKACHE

At the Department of Medical Science, Uppsala University, Sweden, amongst a group of computer operators, Qigong was shown to reduce blood pressure, noradrenaline excretion in urine, and influence the heart rate and temperature, indicating reduced activity of the sympathetic nervous system. Qigong also reduced low-back symptoms.

QIGONG AND THE HEALTH STATUS OF MIDDLE-AGED WOMEN

At The Department of Applied Mathematics in Taiwan, a 12-week Ba Duan Jin Qigong programme was shown to prevent bone loss, which commonly occurs in middle-aged women.

QIGONG AND BLOOD PRESSURE, HEART RATE AND RESPIRATION RATE

At the department of Qi-Medicine, Institute of Biotechnology, Wonkwang University, Iksan, Republic of Korea, heart rate, respiratory rate, systolic blood pressure and rate–pressure product were significantly decreased during Qi training.

QIGONG AND INSOMNIA

At the Qigong Department of Ningbo Hospital of Traditional Chinese Medicine, in China, 76 out of 78 found relief from insomnia using Qigong without the need for drugs.

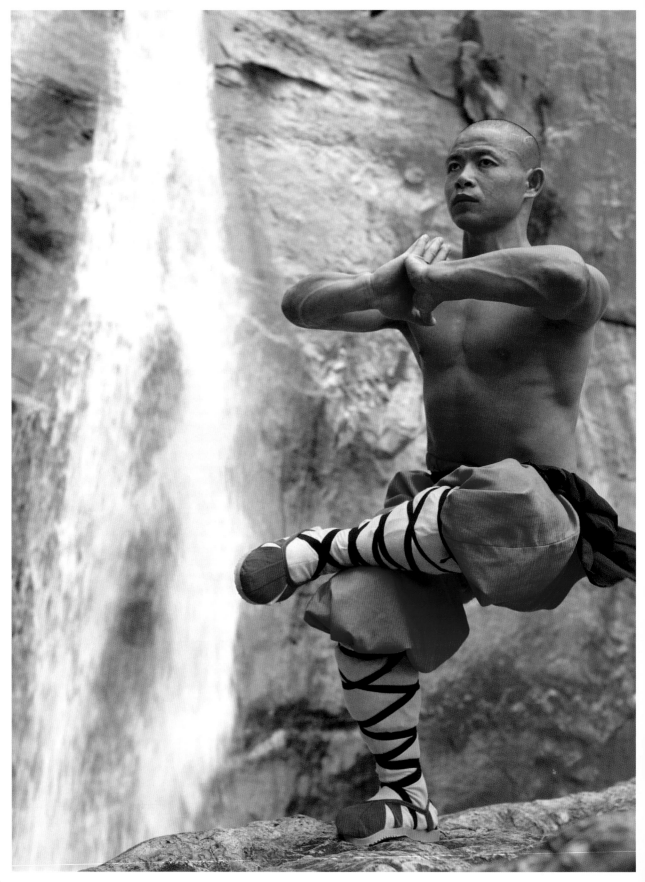

A PRESCRIPTION FOR HEALTH

In general Qigong:

Normalizes blood pressure

Reduces the levels of stress hormones in the blood

Reduces one's biological age

Reduces wear and tear on the body

Helps people to sleep well

Helps people to live longer

Boosts the immune system

Increases feelings of peace and well-being

The reason that Qigong has such a long list of benefits is because it works holistically with the body rather than targeting specific illnesses like we tend to do in the West. Performed correctly there are no side effects and it has both preventative and curative effects.

CHAPTER FOUR

THE SHAOLIN TEMPLE

"A SPECIAL TRANSMISSION OUTSIDE THE SCRIPTURES. NOT DEPENDENCE UPON WORDS AND LETTERS: DIRECT POINTING TO THE HUMAN MIND; SEEING INTO ONE'S OWN NATURE AND ATTAINING BUDDHAHOOD."

Bodhidharma

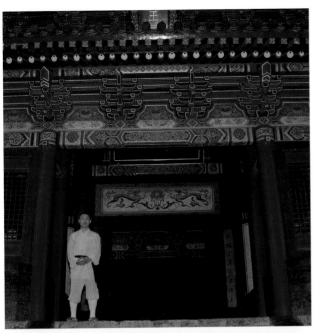
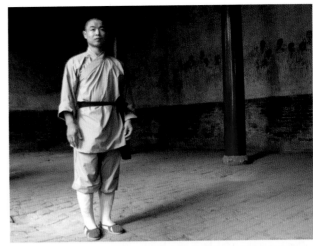
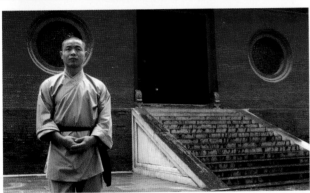
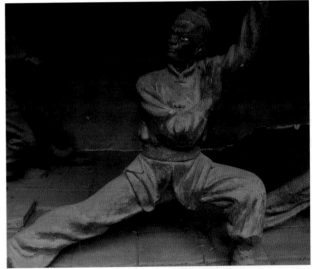
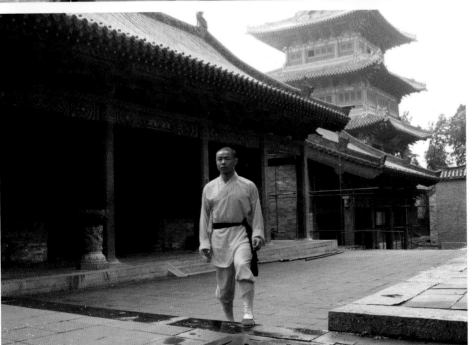
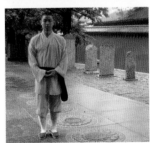
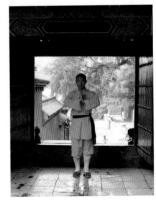

The Qigong that I teach in this book is a Buddhist Qigong from the Shaolin Temple in China. The Shaolin Temple is the birthplace of martial arts and Ch'an Buddhism. An Indian monk called Bodhidharma established Ch'an Buddhism at the Shaolin Temple from where it later travelled to Japan and became known more famously as Zen.

BODHIDHARMA

When Bodhidharma arrived in China in 527 A.D. he found the monks spent most of their time studying the Buddha's teachings in the hope they could gain enlightenment. Bodhidharma felt that reading Buddha's words was as useful as looking at a menu in a restaurant but not eating the food or reading a prescription that the doctor has written but not taking the medicine. This is demonstrated by a conversation Bodhidharma had with Emperor Wu.

Emperor Wu asked, 'What is the most important thing in Buddhism?' Bodhidharma replied, 'There is no such thing.' Emperor Wu then asked, 'Who is standing before me?' Bodhidharma answered, 'I don't know.' Emperor Wu continued, 'How much merit have I earned by ordaining monks, building monasteries and having sutras copied?' Bodhidharma answered, 'None.'

Bodhidharma then crossed the Yangtze River and travelled to the Shaolin Temple where he withdrew into a cave in the mountains and was nicknamed 'The Brahmin Who Stares At The Wall.'

YI JIN JING XI SUI JING

"Bodhidharma travelled to the East to teach these two Yi Jin and Xi Sui classics. A bird like the crane is able to live long, an animal like the fox can be immortal, a human who cannot learn from these classics is worse than the birds and animals."

As well as practising sitting meditation, Bodhidharma discovered that the training of the physical body was just as important as the training of the mind. Without a strong and healthy body enlightenment was impossible to reach. When he emerged from his cave nine years later he taught the monks two Qigong forms that he had created in the cave.

These are called Yi Jin Jing (Muscle/ Tendon Changing Classic), and Xi Sui Jing (Bone Marrow Cleansing Classic). The Shaolin monks who trained in these forms found that not only did the movements increase their health but also they greatly increased their strength. They then began to practise these Qigong forms with Kung Fu and found that this increased their martial power immensely.

Emperors often enlisted Shaolin monks to help them defend their thrones against invaders. As there were no guns or bombs at that time the monks had to use their bodies as weapons. Combining Qigong with Kung Fu made this possible.

BA DUAN JIN

"One should not be governed by Yin and Yang they should use the body of blood and Qi and change it into a body of metal and stone."

A few hundred years later, a monk took eight groups of the most powerful movements from these two forms. This form is called Ba (eight) Duan (best) Jin (movements) or The Eight Treasures. This is the form that is taught in this book.

When my Master transmitted it to me he told me it was one of the most powerful Qigong forms for health. Since coming to the West, I have seen many different interpretations of the Eight Treasures. This version is the Buddhist form that I was taught at the Shaolin Temple, which I have authenticated against the ancient Shaolin books.

Although it is a Buddhist Qigong form, we do not need to be Buddhists to practice the Shaolin arts. People of all religions and those of none practise Shaolin. However knowing a little Ch'an philosophy can help us greatly, not only with our Qigong practice but also with our life.

CHAPTER FIVE

CH'AN BUDDHISM

"YOU MIGHT THINK YOU CAN FIND BUDDHA OR ENLIGHTENMENT SOMEWHERE BEYOND THE MIND BUT NO SUCH PLACE EXISTS"

Bodhidharma

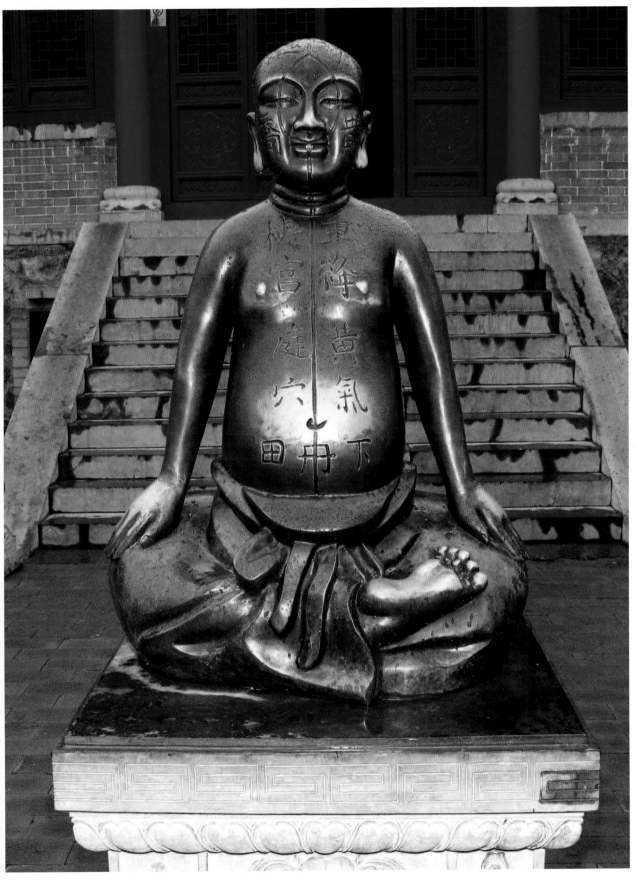

43

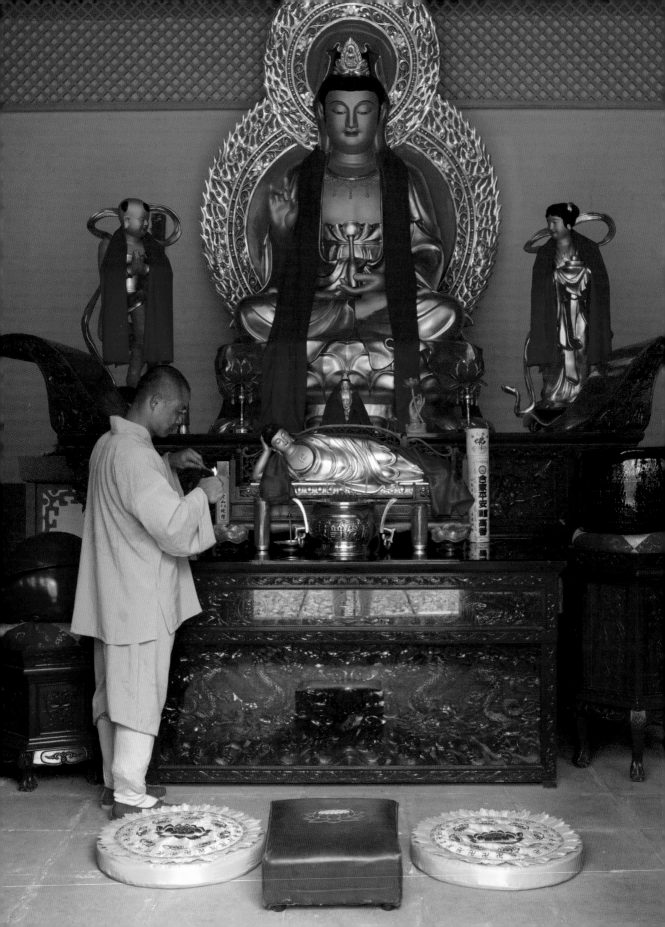

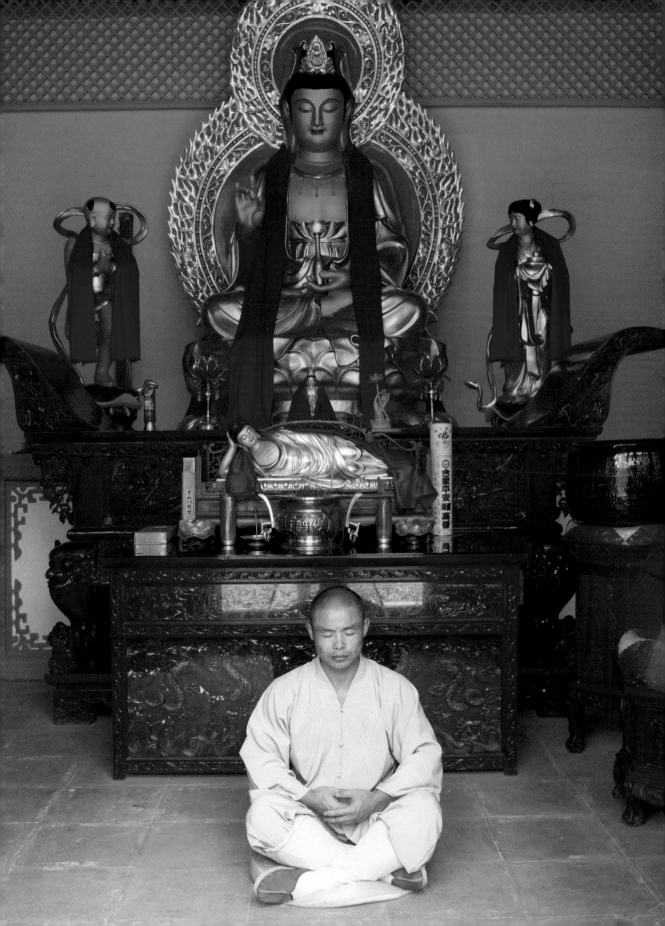

THE ART OF WAR

Many people believe there is a contradiction between learning the art of fighting and being a peaceful Buddhist. In The Art of War, Sun Tzu said,

> *Know thy foe and know thyself: had you a hundred battles to fight you would emerge a hundred times victorious,*
> *Know not thy foe and know thyself: you may lose you may win,*
> *Know neither thy foe nor thyself: every battle you reckon up will be a loss.*

Through the Shaolin Arts we learn about ourselves and through learning about ourselves we learn about life. Our aim is to conquer ourselves not others. The emphasis is always put on the present moment because this is the only time when we are fully alive. We don't practise to be a great martial artist or to lose weight or be healthy or because we think it is good for us, neither do we practise to gain confidence or a sense of peace and harmony or a beautiful body. We may gain all of these but they are the by-products that come from what we do.

Just as a Zen Archer never worries about where the arrow is going to land, we also don't think about what we may gain from our practice. Those thoughts and goals only take us away from the present moment. The point of power is in the now. Now can never be returned to us so we give everything we have to our practice. We concentrate with 100 % of our heart.

MIND HEART NOW

The Chinese character for Mindfulness has two parts, the upper part means 'now' and the lower part means 'heart' or 'mind'. In China we don't separate the mind from the heart the way it is separated in the West. The mind is the heart. The link between our mind and body is our breath. In our Shaolin training we use our breath and movement as an anchor to bring us right here into the now. It's simple. That is all we need to do.

BREATH AND MOVEMENT, MOVEMENT AND BREATH

The only thing to remember when you practise Shaolin is: correct movement, concentrated mind. The mind concentrates on two things; breath and movement, movement and breath. Only when the breath and the movements have become second nature can we gain a deeper awareness of our body.

NO THINKING

The practice is so simple that many people add confusion to it. They start thinking, 'I am breathing and moving,' or they become self-conscious or they may study complex Qi theory and read books on the subject but this only confuses the mind and takes us further away from our own personal experience.

BITE INTO THE APPLE

"It's like when you drink water: you know how hot or cold it is, but you can't tell others."

There is nothing secret, fanciful or complex about Qigong, and the benefits are not just for Shaolin monks but they are within everyone's reach. Personal experience is all that counts. If you are hungry and you haven't eaten for days and I hold up a picture of an apple and tell you about the nutritious benefits of the apple, this won't take away your hunger. Better I give you an apple and you bite into it. Qigong can never be understood consciously just as no one can ever grasp the moon's shadow on the surface of the lake.

INTERDEPENDENCE

Everything in the Universe is interdependent, we take in oxygen and we breathe out carbon dioxide, we eat food and we expel waste products. Through these simple acts we are connected to the Universe. Qigong helps us to go beyond our small individual selves and find a connection with the very fabric of the Universe. It does not give us anything new; it simply connects us with the body's internal power and automatic wisdom that already exists within us.

CHOCOLATE OR QIGONG

In the West we have lost touch with this. If we have a sweet tooth, we generally use our willpower to stop eating chocolate or we may subject ourselves to diets or vitamins, but these are all external methods.

You may be surprised to find that once you start to practise Qigong, these cravings naturally cease and instead you crave healthy food. This happens for a number of different reasons. Chocolate releases endorphins and so does Qigong. Qigong reduces stress. Stress has an effect on the hormonal and endocrine system. An imbalance in the hormones may lead to a craving for sugar or chocolate.

NO EFFORT

Our body has the power to self-regulate itself, without the intervention of diets or medicine or herbs. If we suffer from lower back pain it may disappear, feelings of anxiety will lift, confidence will be regained. All of this will happen without a single effort or thought or desire from you. All you are doing is focusing on the breath and the movement, and the movement and the breath.

YOU ALREADY ARE WHAT YOU WANT TO BECOME

Everything you are,
everything you do,
that's your true mind,
that's your true Buddha.

Bodhidharma

Everything you are looking for is right here. You already are what you want to become. Does a tree have to do something? The purpose of a tree is to be itself, and your purpose is to be yourself. We have everything we need. There is no need to put anything in front of us and run after it. We don't have to add anything extra to ourselves. Right now, we have all the elements for our health. We just have to apply the Shaolin techniques we are learning.

Bringing this energy into our practise gives it a wakefulness that it may not have if we think, "there's something wrong with me," or "I need to go to a mountain to practice" or "tomorrow I won't think so much," or "tomorrow I'll have more time."

Being mindful protects our practice like a candle flame sheltered from the wind.

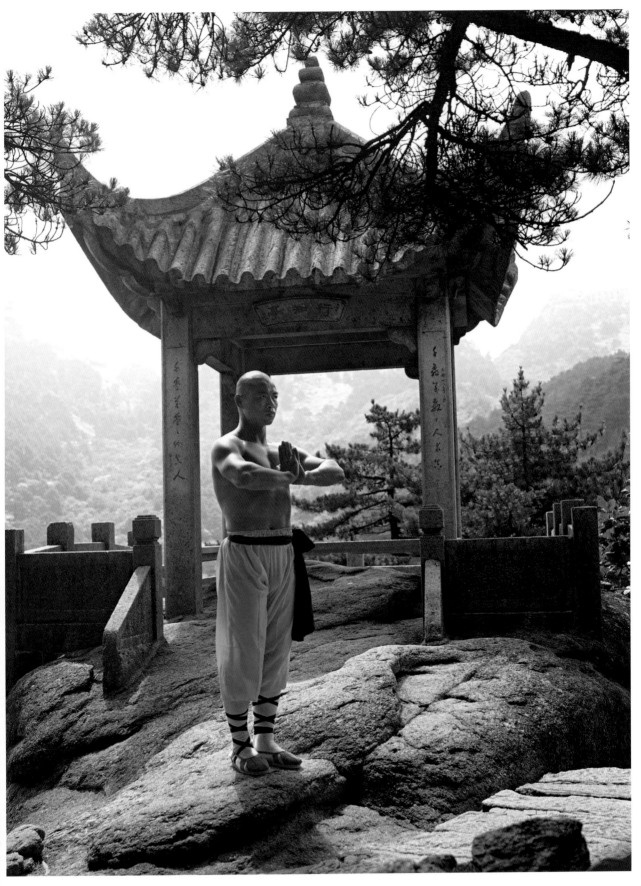

CHAPTER SIX

STEPPING ONTO THE PATH

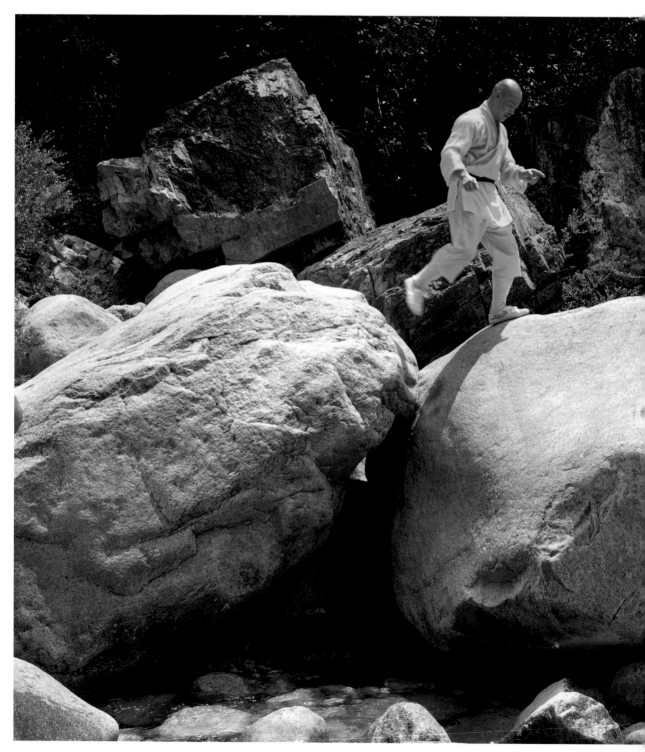

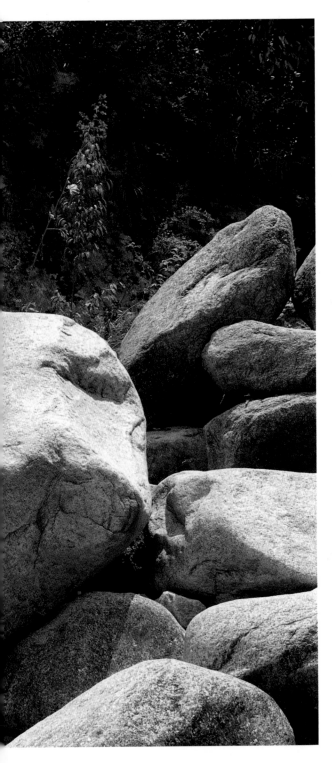

"WHEN YOU
REALIZE
THERE IS
NOTHING
LACKING,
THE WHOLE
WORLD
BELONGS
TO YOU."

Tao

TAKING THE FIRST STEP

This book is not a rigid workout programme but a step-by-step training manual. In the beginning it is important that you don't miss a step, but you follow the book through to the end. You need to know the Shaolin Basics and The Five Fundamental Stances before you learn the Qigong form. Once you understand the basics and have learnt the movements your Qigong routine will consist of four steps:
1) Warm Up
2) Stretching
3) Qigong
4) Qigong Massage

CLOTHING

You don't need any equipment to practise Shaolin Qigong. Wear loose comfortable clothes, preferably made from natural fibres. It's best to wear soft flat shoes. At the Shaolin Temple we wear Feiyue shoes; these are perfect for training as they have flexible soles.

SPACE

The best place to practise is in a place that is free from distractions. In China many people practise in a park but this isn't a necessity. If you don't have access to outside space then turn your mobile off and switch your answer phone on.

Stand up and stretch your arms straight out to the side, then straight out in front of you and finally stretch them above your head. This is how much space you need for your practice. One of the beauties of Qigong is that it can be done anytime and virtually anywhere. As you advance in your practice, external distractions will no longer act as a hindrance and you'll even be able to practise in a crowded place.

TIME

Choose a regular time and stick to it so it becomes a part of your routine and your body expects it as much as it expects you to brush your teeth when you get up in the morning. Making it a part of your routine is the trick to making it a part of your life. Some people prefer to practise first thing in the morning, others in the evening. The key is consistency.

SECRET

When we first start, it is best not to talk about what we are doing to other people at work or when we meet our friends as this can have an effect on our energy and concentration. We may feel excited about our new lease of life and want to share it with others, but it is best to keep our training secret. In this way a more concentrated energy develops.

SIMPLE

Keep the practice simple and set attainable goals for yourself. To get the maximum benefit it is beneficial to train at least three times a week. Write it in your diary so that it is the same time each week. If you are pushed for time, a good trick is to tell yourself you'll do ten minutes. By the time you get to the end of ten minutes you'll probably find that you are enjoying yourself so much that you want to carry on.

If you are unable to commit to so much time then take small steps. While the steps may be small, what you are reaching for is not.

SMALL STEPS TO WELLNESS

Practise the breathing technique when you are driving to work or sitting on the bus or train.

Visualise the form or the five stances when you are waiting in a queue.

Stand straight and grab the floor with your feet at the bus stop.

Start your day with the first exercise from the Eight Treasures.

Get up early one morning a week and do some stretching in your local park.

Stop work and breathe deeply for a few minutes.

Take five minutes each day to do some Qigong.

These small manageable steps will lead to change and this change will increase your desire and confidence to take larger steps so you can embark on a regular Shaolin Qigong Workout.

A NEW SHAOLIN BODY

The photos in this book are meant as both a guide and inspiration. If you haven't done any exercise for a while or you're as stiff as a board, please don't feel discouraged. You will get as much benefit from your

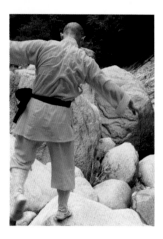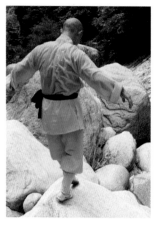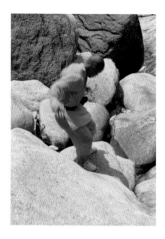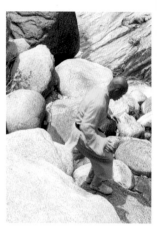

stretch and stance as I do from mine and over time you'll be surprised at how flexible and strong you become. My oldest student is seventy-three and he can testify to that.

It's easy to learn Shaolin and easy to get the benefit. The only thing you need to add to the teachings is time. We believe that it takes three months of regular training to create a healthy Shaolin body. Your eyes will be bright, your skin soft and healthy, your breath deep and stable, your internal organs strong, your muscles flexible.

OPTIMUM HEALTH

If you are training as a martial artist then this is the first stage of your training because without optimum health you cannot progress to the harder practices. These teachings will act as the foundation of your Shaolin training which you will always come back to.

If you are training for health then these teachings are all you will need to maintain good health on the inside and out, together with flexibility, mobility and coordination into your later years. They will help you to get to know your body. The more you know the body, the more you know how far you can push yourself.

STEP BY STEP

Whatever your motivation, you need to build your practice step by step. The beauty of the Shaolin Qigong Workout is that you can easily fit it into your life and it can be varied according to age, health, fitness level or lifestyle.

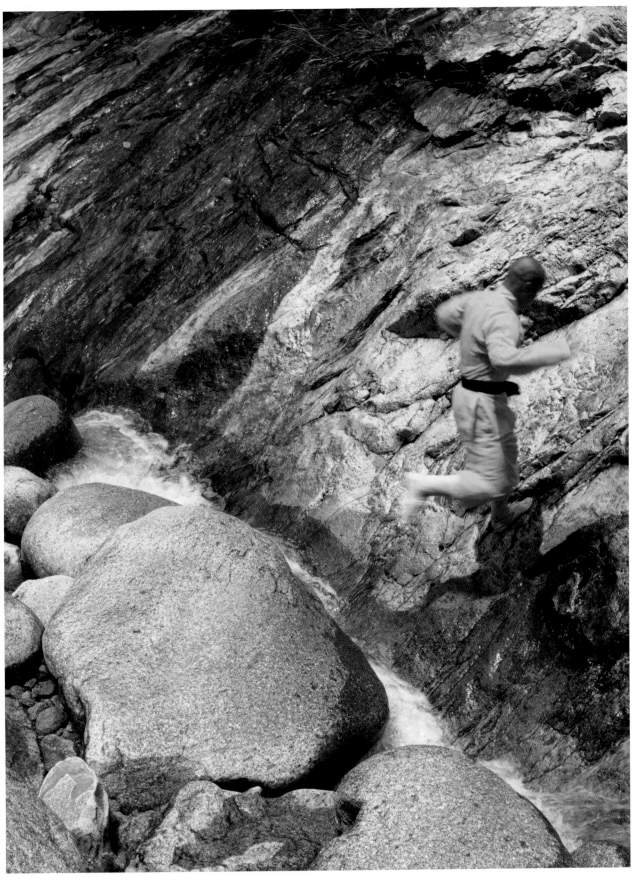

CHAPTER SEVEN

MY JOURNEY TO SHAOLIN

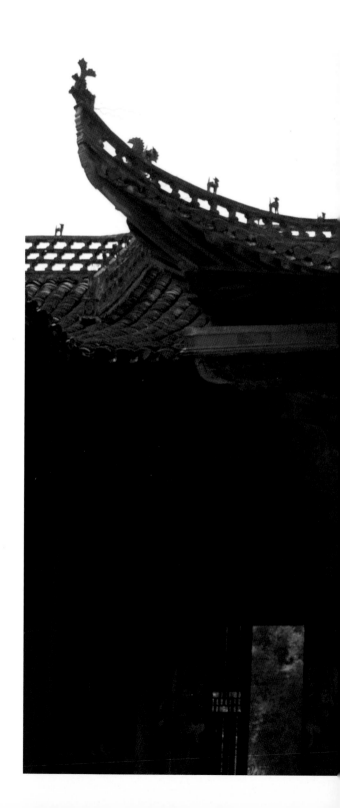

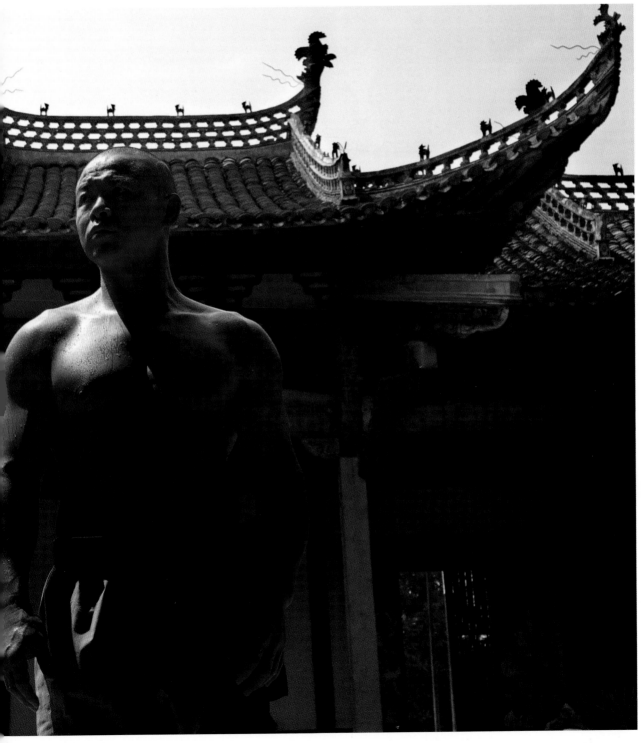

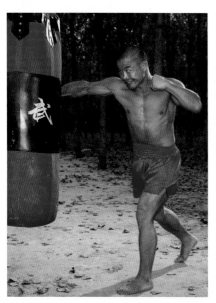
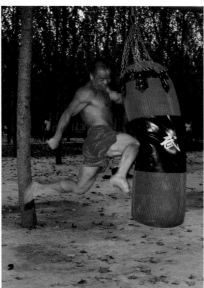
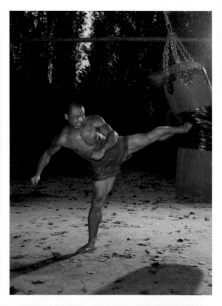
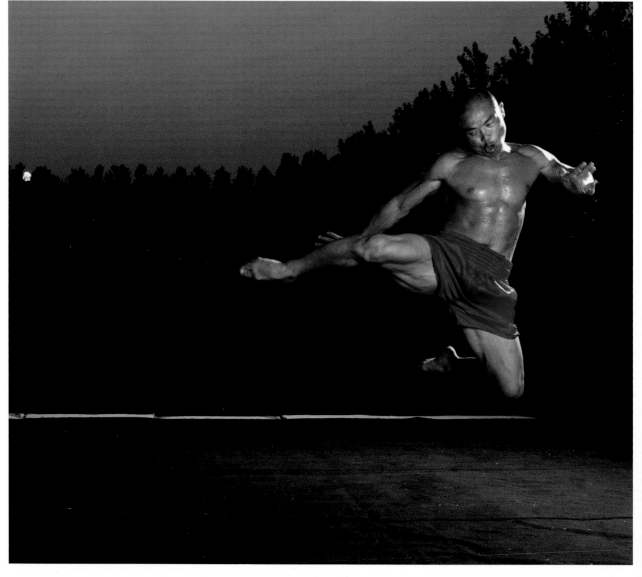

Before you begin on your journey to Shaolin, I would like to share with you a little of how I became a Shaolin Temple disciple.

I come from the largest province in China. Encircled by mountains, Xin Jiang borders on Mongolia, Russia and Pakistan. The population is a mix of Han Chinese and Muslim Uyghur and our food reflects this. We eat spicy lamb, handmade noodles and flat bread made from milk and sesame that we bake in a brick oven. I miss this food now that I live in the West.

Of course, when I was growing up I didn't have access to this abundance of food. Like most people in China, my family were so poor that my parents struggled to feed us. From December through to April our diet consisted of potatoes, carrots, onions and steamed bread. We hardly ever ate fish or meat, and as a child I was used to the constant pang of hunger.

I am the youngest of three brothers and three sisters, which meant that as the political climate began to change, I was the only one in our family who would have the opportunity to go to school and onto university. It took a lot of persuasion before my family let me study at the Shaolin Temple but I was determined.

Because I was the youngest, my brothers were always bullying me, and being the smallest boy in my year meant I also got bullied at school. My dream was to become a great fighter so I would come back to my province a hero and beat up every one that had wronged me.

When I was fourteen I knelt at my father's bed and asked him to allow me to go and train at the Shaolin Temple. When he woke up in the morning I was still there. He didn't say yes or no, but drove me to the station.

I was very excited because I had never travelled by train before. The journey took three days by train and another five hours by bus. When I got to Henan Province everything was new to me. Even the food was totally different to what I was used to. I had never seen a car before, I had never seen so many shops, and I walked around like a tourist taking everything in.

At the temple I shared a room with twenty other boys who were all about my age. At 5.30 am we were woken. We had fifteen minutes to wash and go to the toilet before we lined up at 5.45 and waited for our teacher. We then ran up the Songshan Mountain to the Bodhidharma cave, our feet in rhythm with each other. Once we came back we began our martial training of kicks, stances, jumps, punches and forms.

We were also taught a lot of acrobatics and forms for performance and demonstration. They looked beautiful and impressive but my main motivation was to learn how to fight and this is what I focused on. I think this may be one of the reasons my master — The Shaolin Abbot Shi Yong Xin - gave me the disciple name of Lei, which means thunder.

Outside the temple I began to test the techniques I had learnt against the older boys who had been here longer than me. Sometimes I would get into such big fights that I'd be arrested and held at the local police station. My Master got tired of coming to release me so he sent me to a Ch'an Temple in another province in the hope that I would calm down.

The Abbot in this temple was a remarkable man. He was the only monk who had remained in the temple when the Red Guards had come. They had beaten him and burnt down most of the temple but still he stayed. He struggled to eat and keep warm but now Buddhism was allowed and the temple was beginning to flourish again.

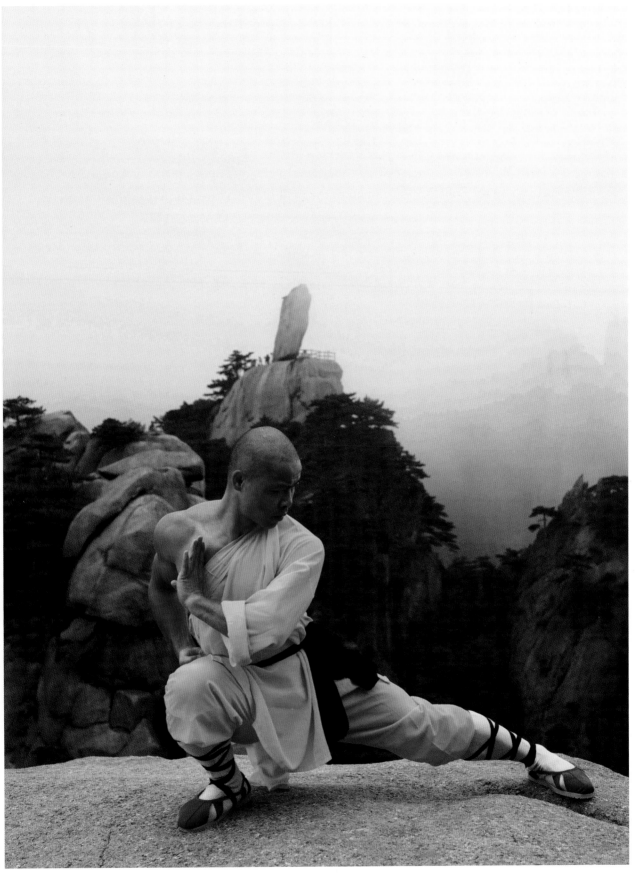

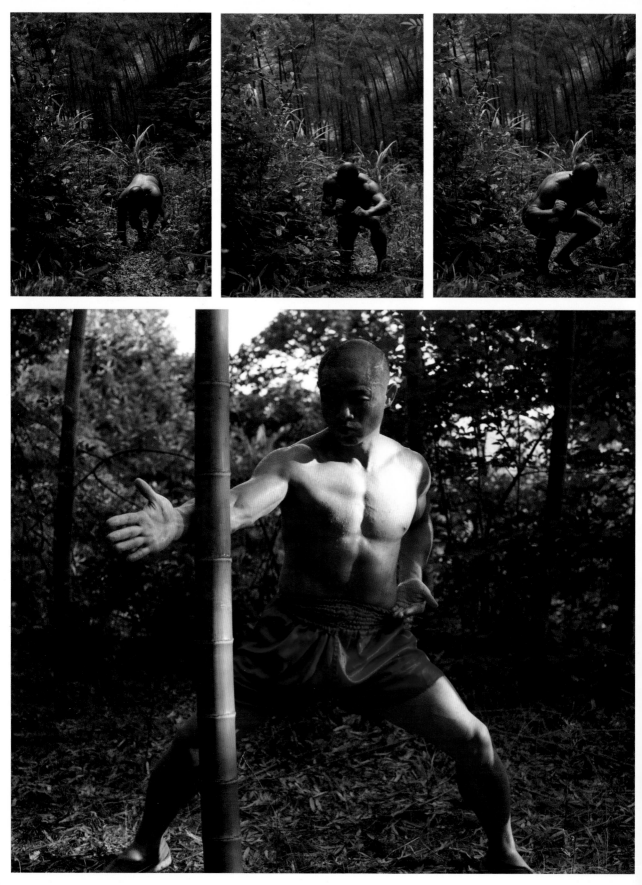

I would go with him when he gave teachings to lay people and in return for the teachings they would offer a donation to help with the cost of re-building the temple. He would wake me in the early hours of the morning and ask me to come and chant with him but I explained to him that I couldn't concentrate. So he asked me what I could concentrate on. I told him: my training. He then instructed me to let my training be my meditation. Just this one sentence changed my life and I suddenly understood why Shaolin martial arts is linked with Buddhism. Through training our body we train our mind.

From that day on, while he chanted I trained. And when I was seventeen he asked me to be ordained as a monk but I told him that I knew nothing about life so how could I become a monk?

At the Shaolin Temple, there are seventy-two different styles and when I returned to the Shaolin Temple my Master told me to specialize in one of them. I decided to choose Shaolin Steel Jacket because I wanted to challenge myself and in some ways, challenge the Shaolin teaching. I had been taught so much performance that I was confused about what was real and what wasn't, and I had to find out for myself.

When people demonstrate Shaolin Steel Jacket, they usually break sticks across their body but this is not real Shaolin Steel Jacket, it is possible to break sticks with muscle alone. Steel Jacket is a fifty - fifty combination of internal and external training, which combines Qigong exercises with intense stamina training and body conditioning. I direct my Qi into my ribs and use bricks or an iron bar to beat myself. My Qi protects my body from injury. But the highest level of Shaolin Steel Jacket is to make our body like a diamond so that disease cannot penetrate.

As I have got older, I've found another way to practise Shaolin Steel Jacket with more of a focus on health and fitness than martial power. I'm still interested in fighting and I coach fighters because I believe it's good for a young person to be challenged in the ring; many young people seem lost and the discipline can give direction to their life and help them to contribute more fully in our society. But I also focus on what is useful for health and fitness. What is the quickest way to instant health and fitness?

The reason I ask this question is because I don't want to waste my time or my student's time. I want to teach them skills that are useful for their life, whether that is fighting stress and fitness levels or fighting an opponent in the ring. Both of these are challenges and we need to cultivate the energy of a warrior to succeed.

After I left the temple, I travelled to other martial arts schools both to learn from different masters and teach what I had learnt at the Temple. In 2000, I was asked by my brother Shifu Shi Yan Zi to come to London and help set up the first Shaolin Temple in Europe. The Abbot was concerned about the spread of un-authentic Shaolin teachings so he wanted a Shaolin Temple in the UK. Up until that time, Shifu Yan Zi and I had only taught students who trained full-time, so we had to find a way to condense the teachings into two hours.

Seeing that Shaolin was having a positive effect on our students which went way beyond the health benefits, I went on to make a series of Shaolin Warrior DVDs so I could share with as many people as possible the true teachings from the Shaolin Temple.

When you step onto the path of Shaolin, you are taking on a tradition which is thousands of years old. Shaolin contains The Tao, Confucius and Ch'an Buddhism; this is why I decided to shoot the photographs in this book in China. I wanted to return to the roots of martial arts and demonstrate the origins of the teachings. They come from the mountains, the bamboo forests, the rice fields and the traditional villages of China. It is this landscape that has given the forms their shape.

Today the majority of us practise in an urban environment. Many of my students are now based in London, New York, Paris and Beijing. As China has prospered, so have they. When my Chinese students came to visit me at the temple, they thanked me for teaching them Shaolin as it has given them the determination, confidence and willpower to succeed as successful businessmen.

I am not a great martial artist which is why I'm always training and always learning. I am not the greatest teacher but I try to give a taste of what Shaolin really is. It's not a dream or a fantasy like it is sometimes made out to be, but the art and science of true health and happiness.

I believe there are no bad students: there are just bad teachers, and if you choose to study from my books then you become my student and I hope I will teach you well.

As you can see from my story I am not a perfect person. The Buddha's flower is the lotus and it grows from mud. Whatever place you are in right now, whatever problems or difficulties you may have, you can use these problems to grow something beautiful through the guidance of the Shaolin teachings. My mud was my poverty and anger; this enabled me to grow as a martial artist. My motivation was naïve but as Shaolin changed me, my motivation also changed.

This series of books is a culmination of my twenty years experience of martial arts and the wisdom that I have learned under the instruction of many great masters. Any errors made are not those of my masters or the Shaolin Temple, but my own.

Yan Lei with his master,
The Shaolin Abbot Shi Yong Xin

PART TWO
THE FUNDAMENTALS OF SHAOLIN QIGONG

CHAPTER EIGHT

COMPLETE QIGONG BREATHING

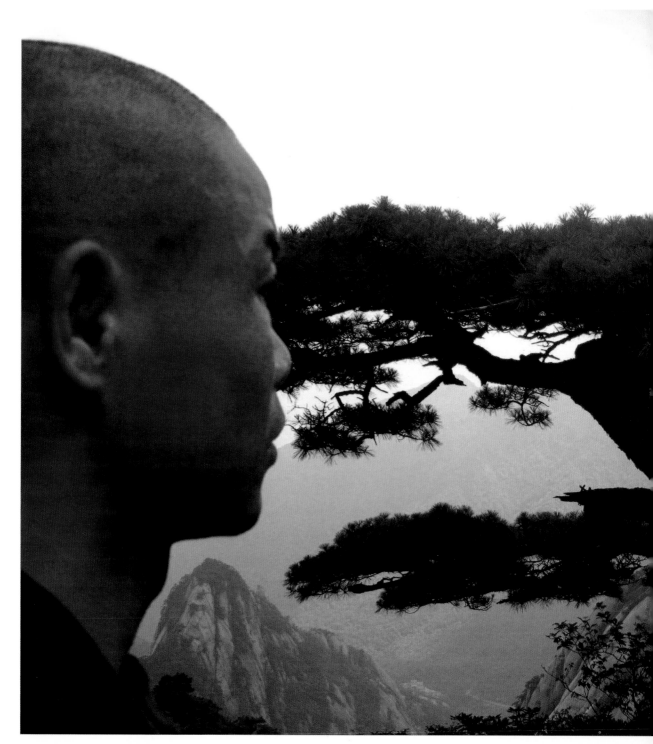

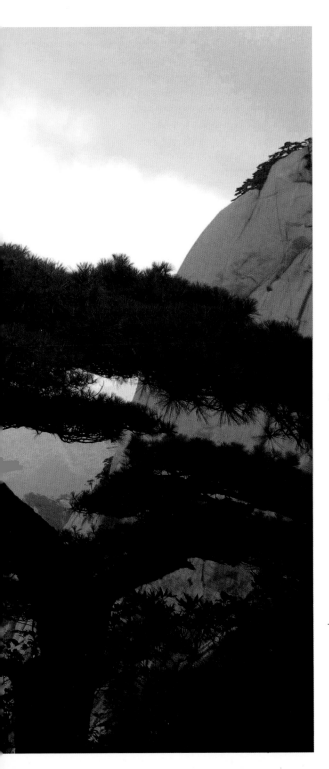

THE LINK BETWEEN MIND AND BODY IS THE BREATH

When you practise Qigong your focus needs to be narrow and rest only on the breath and the movement together. The qualities of these two elements demonstrate the level of your concentration. As your practice deepens, so does your concentration, so that eventually Qigong becomes a meditation in its own right.

Use your nose to inhale and exhale. This is because the nose contains fine hairs that help filter out pollutants and germs; also the air is warmed by the blood flowing through the nose. Your mouth should be relaxed and slightly open with your tongue touching the roof of your mouth. This activates one of the meridians and allows the Qi to circulate. It also stops the throat from getting dry. If any saliva comes into your mouth then swallow it. This makes the Qi travel. At the Shaolin Temple we say if the saliva goes to your heart then it thins your blood, if it goes to your liver then you see things clearly, if it goes to your lungs it makes your Qi stronger, your stomach it helps you to digest, your kidneys it creates more Yang energy. We believe that the saliva goes where the body needs it most.

Oxygen nourishes and replenishes every cell in your body and the simple act of improving your breathing can make a dramatic difference to your overall health and energy level. Our brain uses 20 per cent of our body's available oxygen and deep breathing can help to nourish it. When your breath is deep and relaxed, it's easier to stay calm, grounded and focused on the present moment.

Most people use their chest to breathe, but when we practise Qigong we use the diaphragm. Using your diaphragm deepens your breath and increases the volume of oxygen into your body.

NATURAL ABDOMINAL BREATHING

If you are not used to breathing with your diaphragm and abdomen, then begin by placing your left hand on your side, just below your chest and your right hand on your abdomen. Inhale - but instead of inhaling into your chest, inhale into your diaphragm. Feel your diaphragm and abdomen expand and push against your hands. Now, exhale and feel your diaphragm contract and your abdomen suck in. Try again - when you inhale, your diaphragm and abdomen expands, and when you exhale, your diaphragm and your abdomen contracts.

Check that your shoulders are relaxed and that your mouth and tongue haven't tensed up. When you inhale, there should be no rising of the shoulders and very little movement in the chest.

It may feel strange at first but this is your original breath, it's how you used to breathe when you were a child. It's a good idea to get into the habit of breathing with your abdomen rather than your chest because it's the most efficient and healthy breath for day-to-day life.

When we practise Qigong we reverse the direction of our abdomen.

THE BREATH OF QI

This breathing technique helps us to get the maximum benefit from our practice. It is not a natural way to breathe, so it is not how we would breathe when we are going about our normal activities. Reversed abdominal breathing is used solely for Qigong and it can also be used for sitting meditation to help to clear and energize the mind.

Usually when we inhale, our stomach expands and when we exhale it contracts, but with the breath of Qi, we do the opposite. When we inhale our stomach contracts and the air goes into our lungs and chest, and when we exhale our stomach expands.

Begin by placing your left hand on your side, just below your chest and your right hand on your abdomen. Inhale - this time your diaphragm will contract and your abdomen will contract, at the same time your chest will expand. Exhale - your diaphragm and stomach will expand. Make sure your shoulders don't rise and fall and that you're not just breathing shallowly into your chest. If you are practicing correctly you will feel an expansion in the lungs and your breath will naturally deepen and lengthen.

Although this method of breathing will feel strange at first, it is important to get it right. Once you have mastered the breathing, you can then pull in the perineum on the inhale and when you exhale relax the perineum. Don't pull it in 100 % as this creates tension in the body, just pull in a little. If you are a total beginner then you don't need to do this until you have fully mastered the breathing and the movement.

An experienced practitioner will make no sound on the inhale and the exhale and this is our aim. Your breath needs to be soft, even, deep, and have a natural flow to it. The most important thing is not to use any energy when you breathe. Many students make the mistake of pushing or holding the breath. This is incorrect, the breath knows how long it can last and there is no need to control it. You also might feel that you can't take enough breath in, this is why we pause for three breaths between each main Qigong movement, so you can regulate and connect with your breathing before continuing with the next move.

Our breathing is the barometer for what is going on in our mind and body; it changes texture and rhythm when we are sad, stressed or relaxed. Through the practice of Qigong we surrender ourselves to the breath and the movement and it naturally calms, deepens and lengthens of its own accord. Once we have truly mastered the breath we will feel as if we are neither inhaling nor exhaling and the breath will enter and leave the body without us being conscious of it. Be aware of your breathing but make sure you give your breath space to breath.

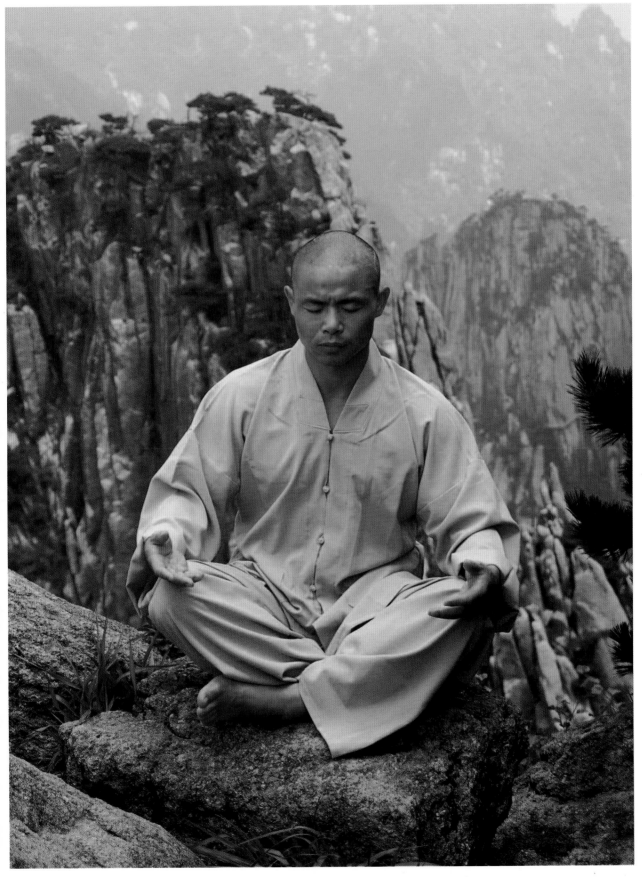

LET THE
BREATH
BREATHE
ITSELF

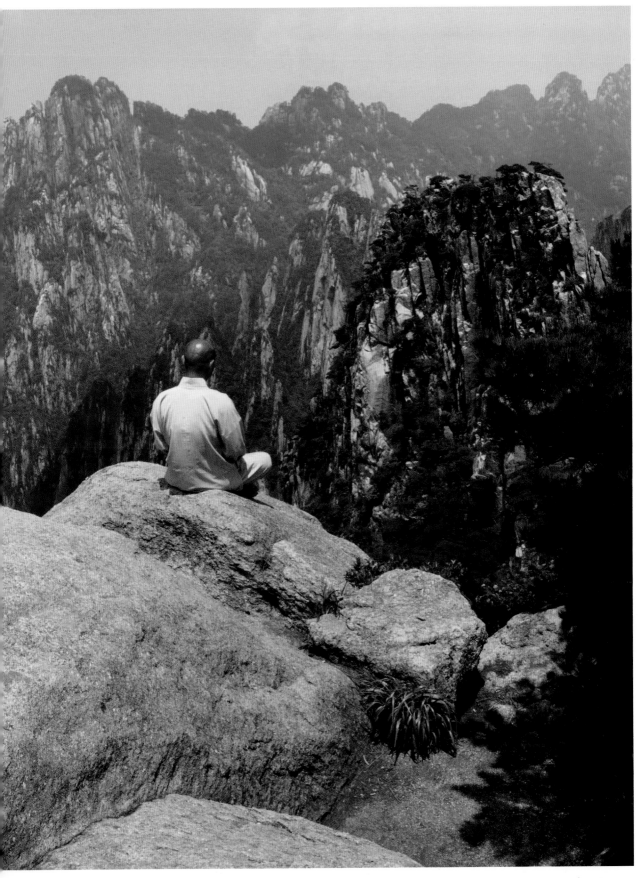

CHAPTER NINE

POSTURE AND MIND

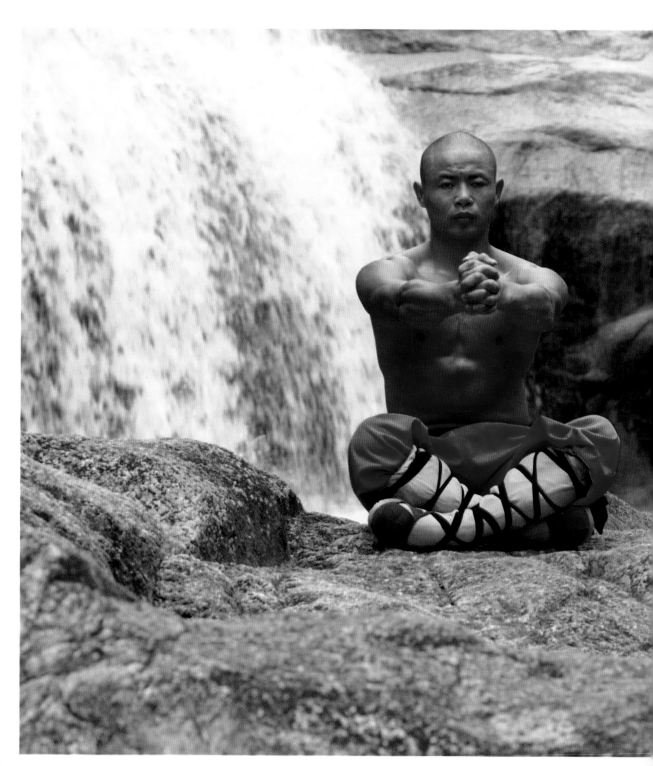

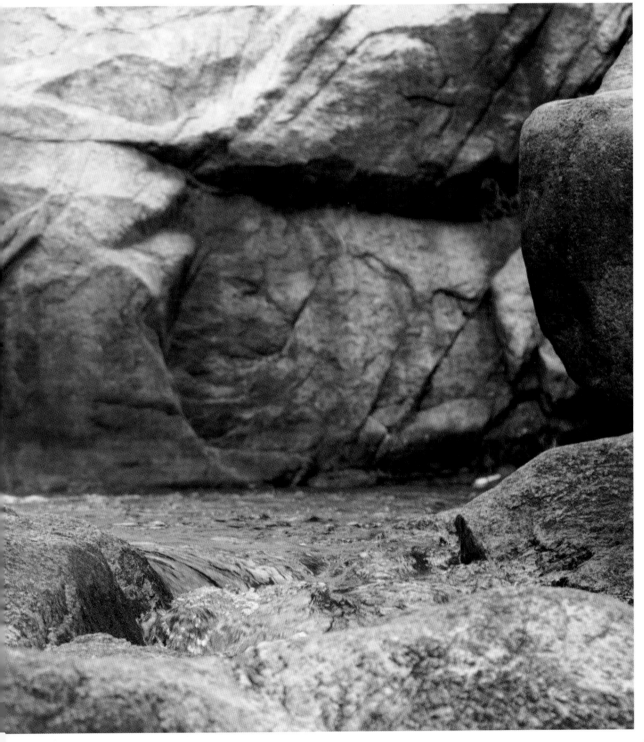

POSTURE

The body is relaxed but not lazy, straight but not stiff. If the spine is bent or crooked then the Qi cannot flow properly.

To lengthen the spine, imagine that your head is suspended from above as though a string were attached to the crown, roll your hips slightly forward so there is a gentle tucking in of the pelvis. Open your chest a little and keep your shoulders down and relaxed. Check that your knees are straight but not locked. Feel the weight of your body evenly on both feet.

Think of a tree – a tree is not tense but is stable and grounded.

Whether we do Qigong or Kung Fu, our feet always grab the floor but they do so in a natural way. At first it will feel tense and unnatural but over time your body will find a relaxed way of doing this. The state of our posture has a surprising effect on our mind. Simply standing straight can help to increase positive feelings.

MIND

It is important that when we begin our training, we focus completely on what we are doing and let go of any worries or concerns we may have. Worries circle in our mind, and the more we think, the more momentum our worries gain. The Shaolin Qigong Workout acts as a pair of scissors, cutting through our thoughts and giving our mind and body a place of refuge and stillness.

We know how energised we feel when we come back from holiday; we can get a taste of that everyday by giving ourselves a holiday from our thoughts. The more we practise, the easier it will become to access this peaceful state of being.

Begin by dedicating this time to your practice. If your mind is full of thoughts, you don't need to resist them as this will make them stronger, but gently let them go. As you continue, your thoughts will naturally quieten down of their own accord.

There is a famous story about one of Buddha's disciples called Shravana. He was a very good guitar player but was having trouble meditating, so he went to the Buddha to ask for advice. The Buddha asked Shravana,

'Does the sound of the guitar come from tight strings or loose strings?' Shravana replied, 'Neither, it is produced by balancing the strings.' The Buddha said, 'It is the same with the mind. The way to meditate is by being tight and relaxed."

And this holds true for your Qigong Workout. It is important to approach your training with the right attitude so that your mind is working with your body rather than opposing it. As beginners, we tend to be more tight then relaxed but over time we learn the correct way to practise.

At the Shaolin Temple, we say that a beginner has five hearts and as you progress with your practice, these five hearts become one.

CHAPTER TEN

FIVE HEARTS

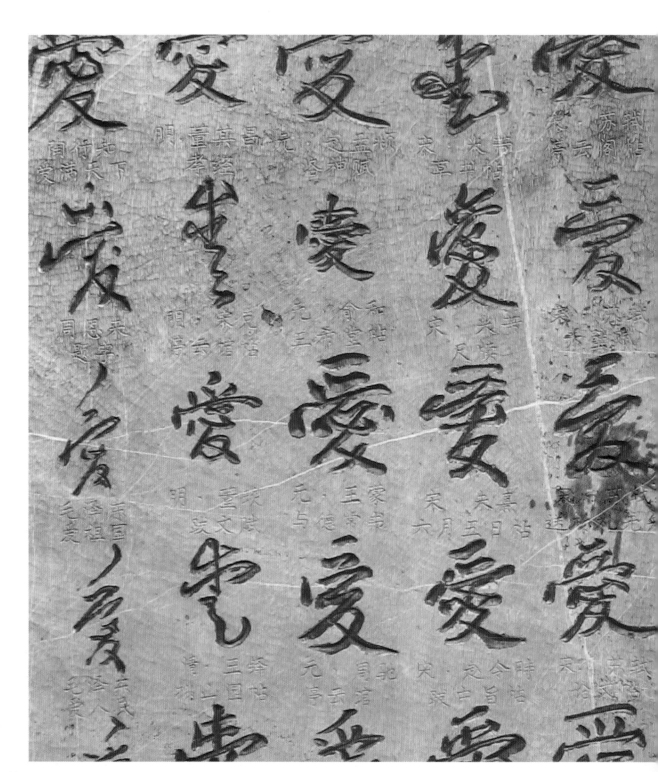

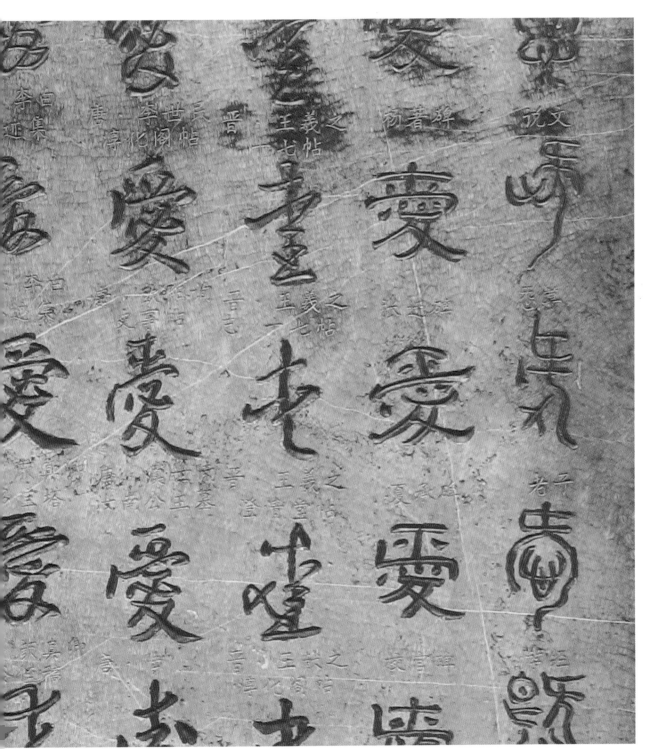

THE HEART OF BELIEF

"Use your mind and heart to believe."

When you practice Shaolin, you need to believe that these exercises can help you. If you don't believe these teachings can help you then it is best not to do them. Faith is like a seed from which positive things can grow, but if faith is not there it is as if the seed is burnt and therefore nothing can grow.

THE HEART OF CONCENTRATION

"Focus mind and heart with body."

Your mind is like a monkey, train it to focus on the breath and the movement. Don't allow your concentration to be coloured by a desire for a feeling in the practice. And when you do have a feeling, don't get carried away by pride. Any effort in your practice should be directed from achievement to non-achievement.

THE HEART OF LOYALTY

"Be loyal to your practice. Use your willpower to develop belief and focus."

In the beginning, your faith may be weak but if you stay loyal to your practice and use your willpower to keep going your faith will strengthen.

THE HEART OF PEACE

"Make your mind and body peaceful so you can understand yourself. Enjoy yourself without desire."

Emotions change the rhythm of breathing. Think about how you breathe if you are angry or anxious. If you are peaceful, then your breathing will be natural and even, and the peaceful nature of your practice will spread like water into all aspects of your life. At the same time, if your actions in your day-to-day life are not peaceful then this too will spread into your practice.

THE HEART OF SKILL

"Become everything you do. Enjoy the moment."

In the beginning, your practice will yield little and you will not have much feeling, but after a while your body will start to have a feeling and it is then that you need to recognise this and use your mind and body together to realize how to cultivate it. The aim of practice is to gain a deeper understanding of yourself.

"Let your life become a meditation."

PART THREE
THE QIGONG WORKOUT FOR LONGEVITY

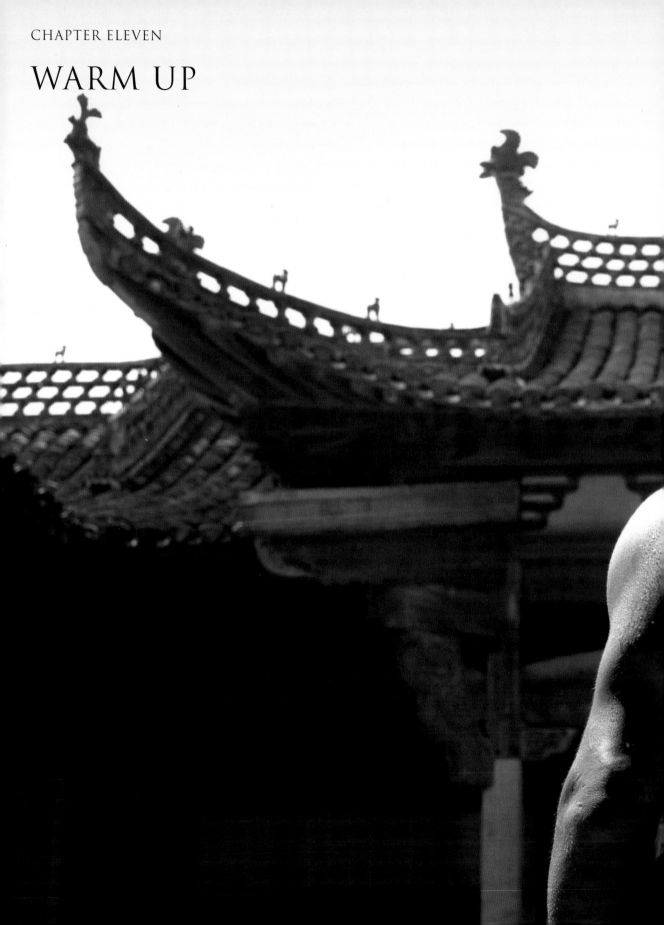

CHAPTER ELEVEN

WARM UP

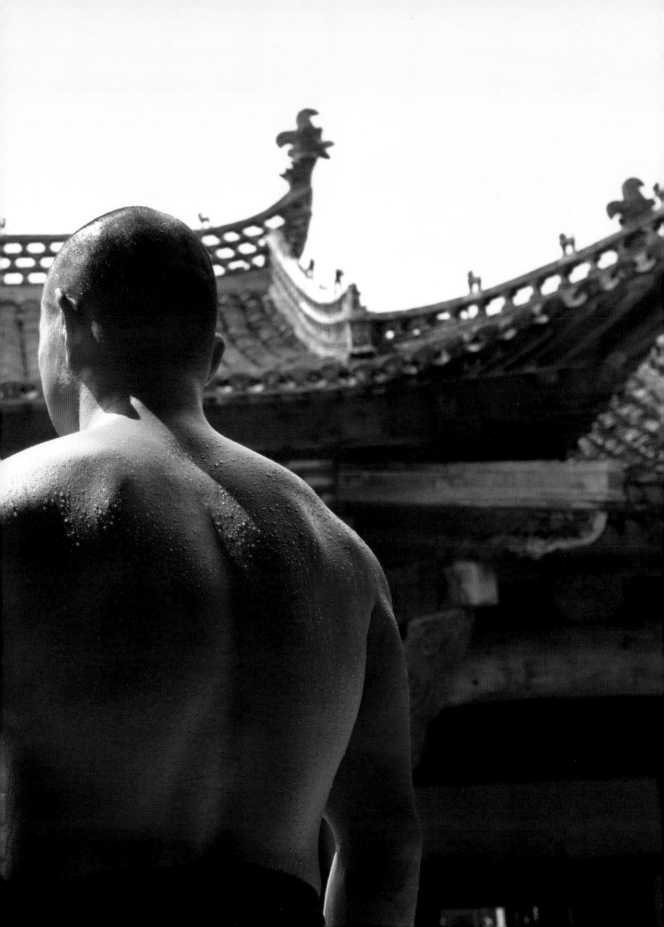

These exercises are not things we learn or do, they are what we are. Try to let go of impatience and wanting to achieve anything, and use the time you do these exercises as time out from the pressure of modern day living and a time to give something back to yourself.

There should be no pain when you do any of these exercises. If there is then stop immediately because you are either doing something incorrectly or you have an injury which means these exercises are not correct for you at this time. Take it gently, don't push yourself, especially in the morning when your muscles and joints will be at their stiffest. Listen to your body and gently build up your flexibility. It is important to do the movements correctly and not force any movements.

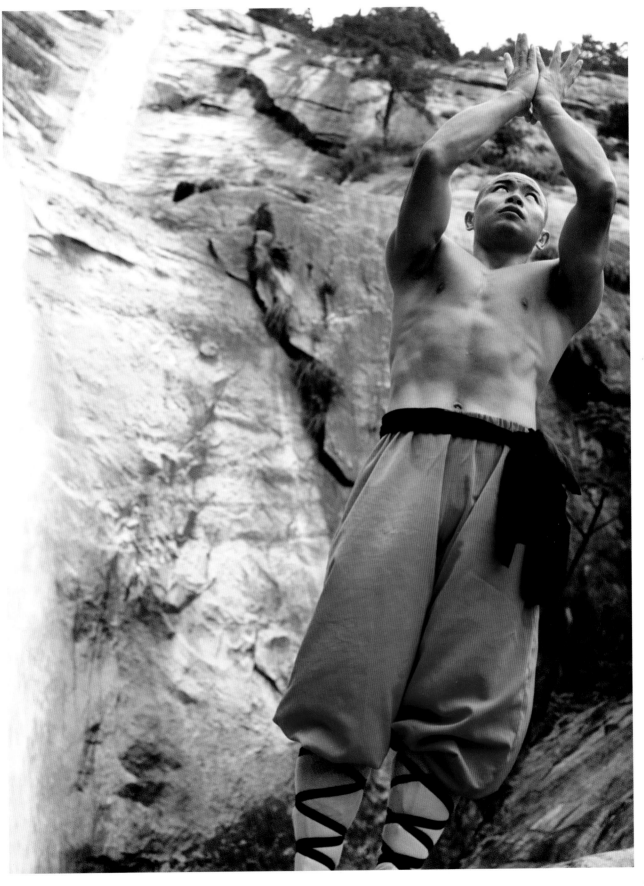

WARM UP

If we are about to embark on a long motorway journey, we usually check our car to make sure there's enough air in the tyres, and oil and water for the engine to run smoothly. At the Shaolin Temple, we check that our joints are okay before we begin our training. The warm up helps to protect us from injury and it is also a time when we can tune into our body and see which parts of the body feel stiff, tense or less flexible.

When we start to warm up, we take it slowly and focus on the part of the body that we are warming up. The warm up exercises usually take between four to seven minutes. Younger people can warm up in four minutes but if you are older, stiffer or haven't done any exercise in a while, you will need to take the full seven minutes.

LABEI
BACK STRETCH

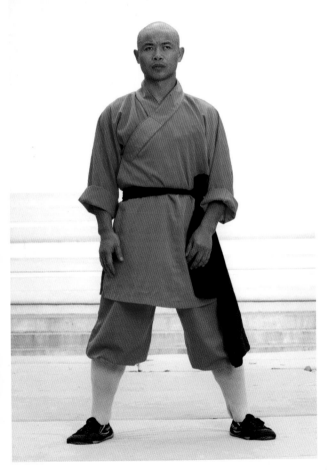

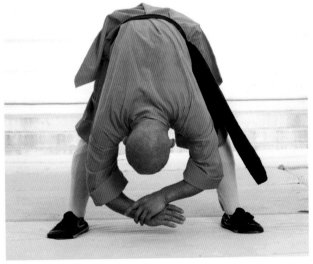

1) Open your feet hip width apart.

2) Drop your head onto your chest and fold forward vertebra by vertebra. Stretch down to the middle of your body and place your left hand over your right hand. Very gently bounce three times in the centre then the left and the right.

REPEAT x3 TO THE CENTRE AND EACH SIDE

Make sure the knees stay straight and the neck and shoulders dropped and relaxed. Your head should be like a rag doll. Check for any tension in your jaw. From this movement go straight into:

SHUAN YAO
WAIST CIRCLE

The aim is to make a complete circle with your upper body. This can be done at a speed which feels right for your body. When we are warming up for Qigong we do this exercise slowly but when we are warming up for Kung Fu we speed this movement up.

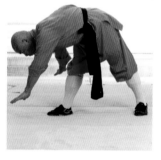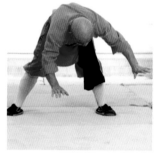

1) – 6) Open your arms and circle your body from the right to the left, continue to circle your body up to the upper left, the centre of the back, the upper right and then down to the lower right.
REPEAT x3
CLOCKWISE AND
3 ANTI-CLOCKWISE.
Your eyes always follow your arms. When you fold forward, you can bend the knees a little, when you stretch up and back, straighten your legs and feel a stretch in your back.

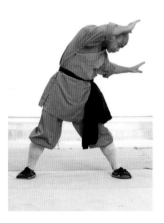 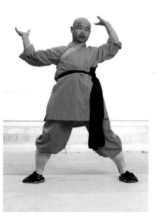 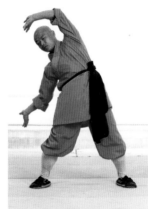 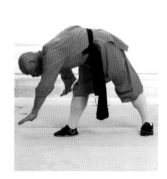

GONG BU LA JIAN
SHOULDER STRETCH

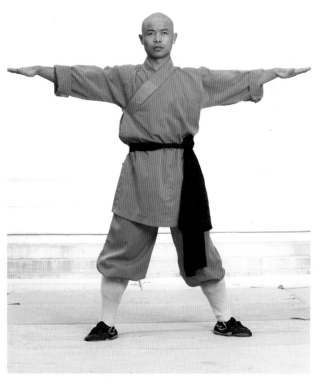

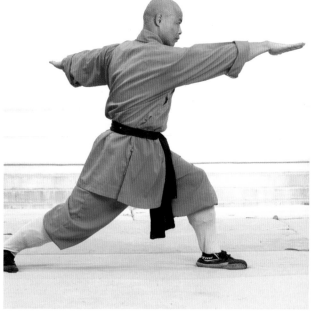

1) Open your feet slightly wider than your hips and take both arms out to the side. Keep your arms straight.

2) Turn to the left and bend your left knee slightly. Keeping your right leg straight, stretch your right arm in front and your left arm behind you.

3) Stretch your arm forward four times then turn to the other
side and repeat.
REPEAT x3 EACH SIDE.

Feel a stretch in your shoulder and keep your arms as straight as possible.

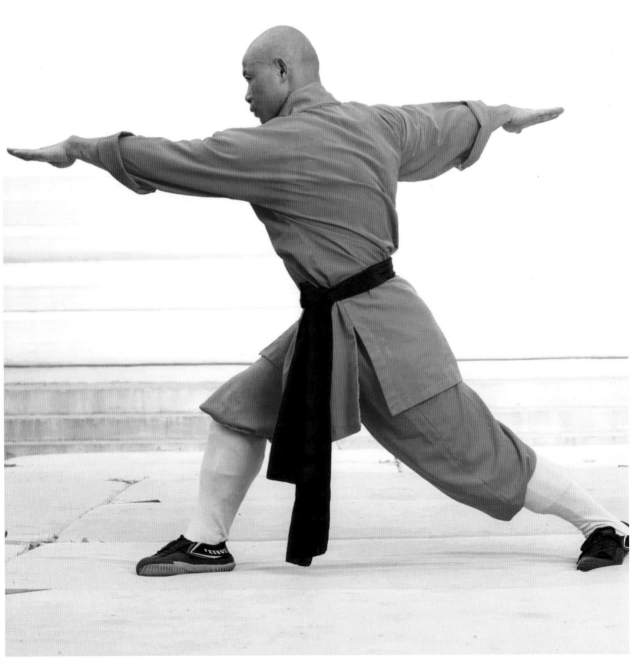

QIAN HOU FU YAO
WAIST WARM UP

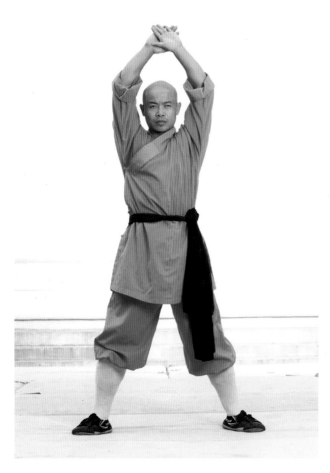

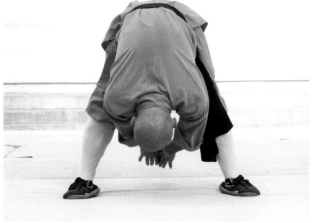

1) Open your feet hip width apart and bring your arms over your head. Place your left hand over the right hand.

2) Bend your waist and place your hands as far as possible through your legs. Gently bounce 3 times.

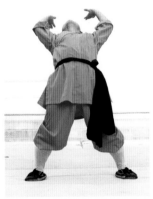

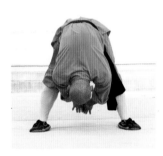

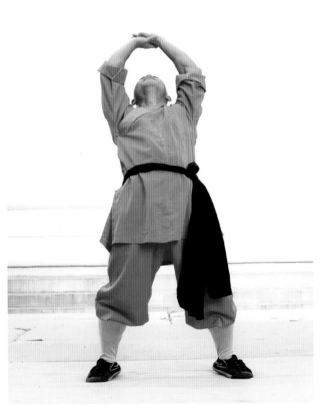

4) Gently bounce 3 times.

5) Bend at your waist.
REPEAT STEPS 2-3 x3

3) Bring your torso upright, bend your legs slightly and stretch your back until your eyes look at the wall behind you.

NECK CIRCLE

With the following exercises the emphasis is on making a circle with each of your body parts that you warm up.

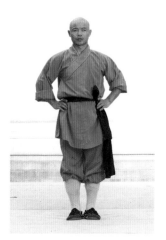 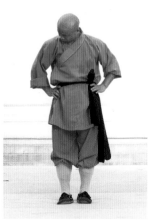 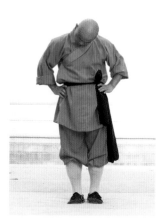 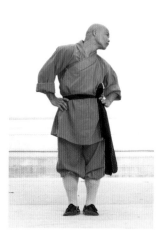

1) – 5) Close your feet, close your teeth, drop your shoulders and slowly circle your neck to the left. Let it follow your natural range of movement, inhaling as you begin moving from the back and to the right.
REPEAT x3 EACH DIRECTION.
Make sure you are only moving your neck for this exercise and not your shoulders or your upper body.

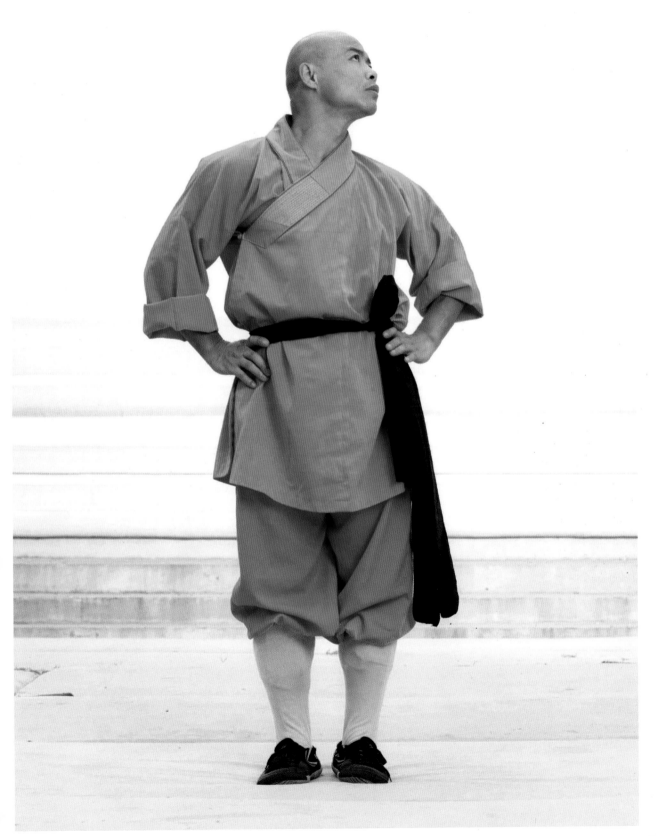

SHOULDER CIRCLE

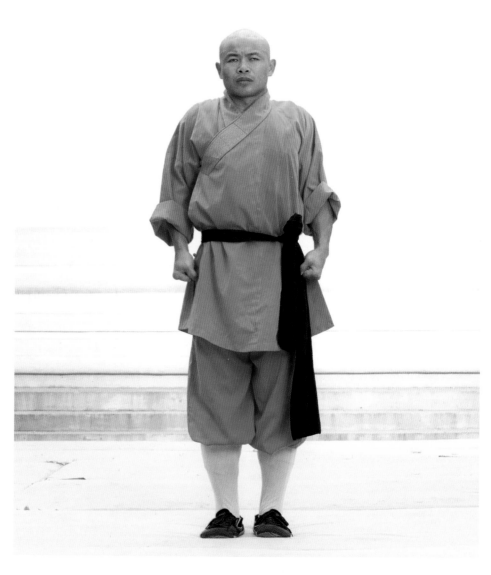

1) Stand straight. Clench your fists and make a circle with your shoulders in a clockwise direction.
REPEAT x3

2) Change sides and circle your shoulders in an anti-clockwise direction.
REPEAT x3

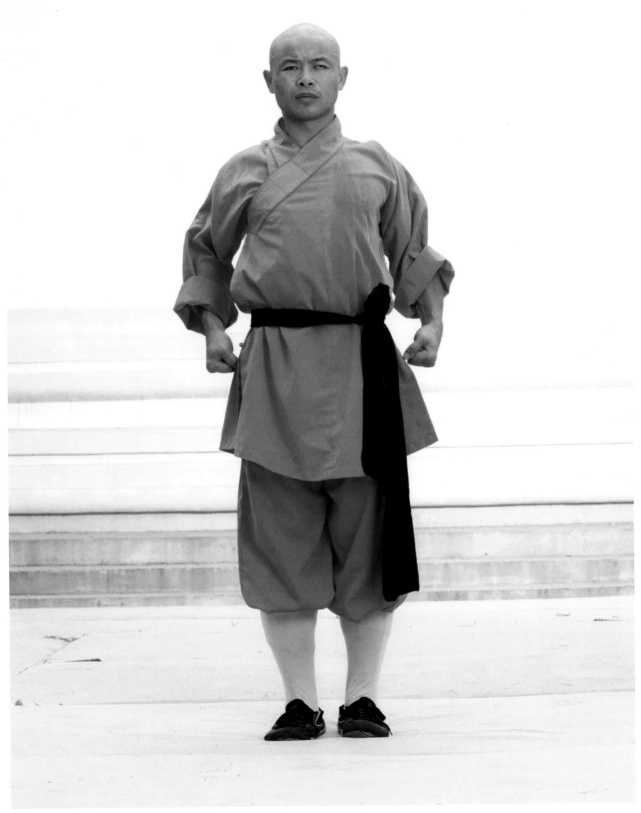

ELBOW CIRCLE

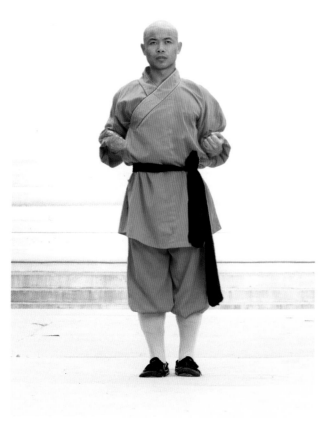
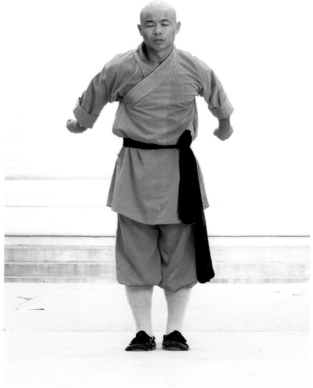

1) Clench your fists. Bend your elbows and draw your fists to your waist until your elbows can't go back anymore. Feel your chest open.

2) Turn your fists into your body and stretch your arms behind your back – feel a stretch in your arm.

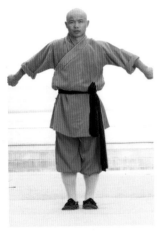 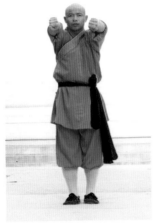 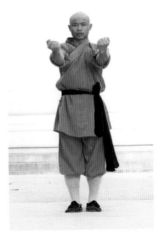 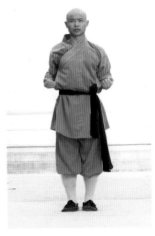

3) 4) Keep your arm straight and circle your arms to the side and then the front of your body – your knuckles should be facing inwards.

5) Turn your fists so your knuckles are facing the ground.

6) Bring your fists back to your waist.
REPEAT STEPS 1-6 x 3

WRIST CIRCLE

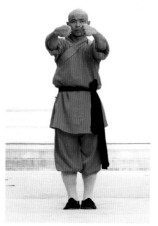 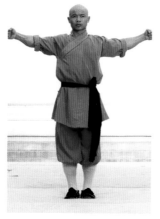 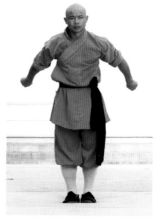 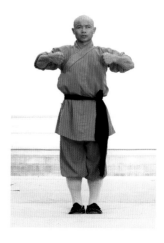

1) Clench your fists and stretch both arms straight out in front of you with your elbows pointing outwards. Bend your fists inwards until you feel a stretch in the wrist.

2) Take both arms out to the side so your shoulders and arms are in one line and your chest feels expanded.

3) Keep moving your arms until they are behind your body. When they can't go back any further...

4) 5) Bring your fists to your chest then push your fists straight out in front of you.

REPEAT STEPS 1-5 x3
The focus is on turning your wrist and feeling a stretch in your wrist.

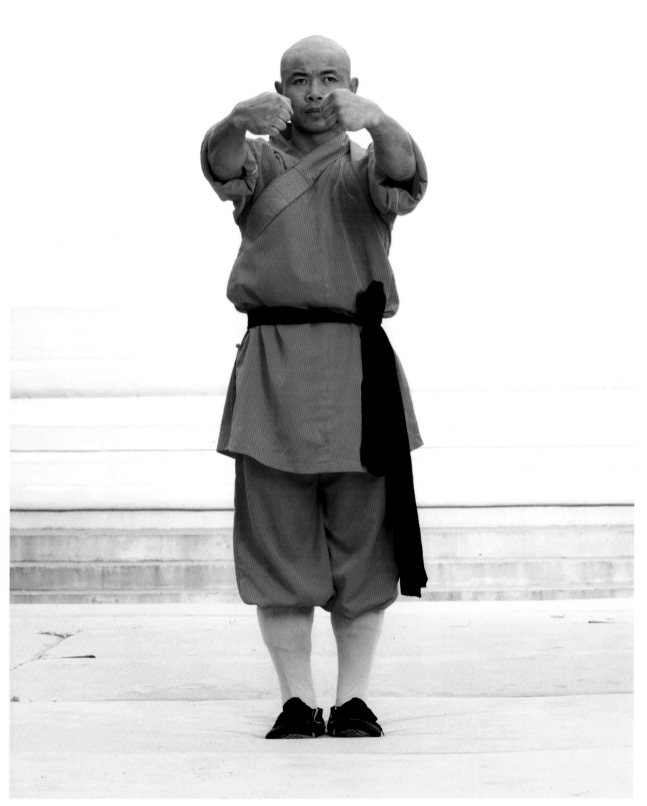

KNEE CIRCLE

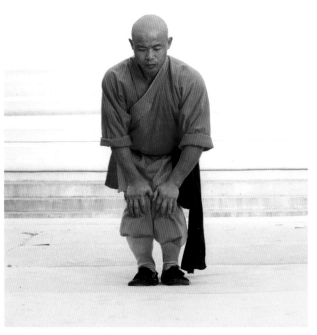 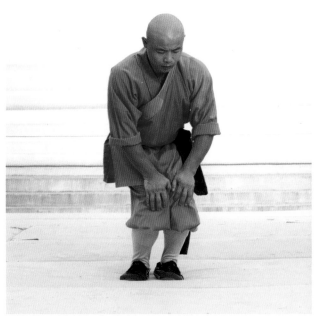

1) – 2) Bend your knees making sure to keep your back straight. Place your hands on your knees and move your knees in a circle from left to right then change direction. REPEAT x3 IN EACH DIRECTION.

ANKLE CIRCLE

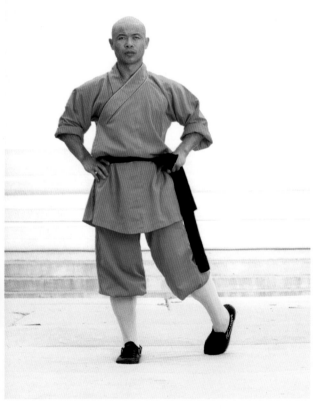 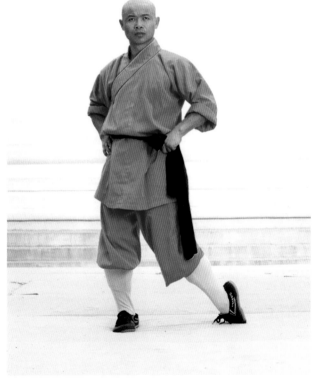

1) Balance on one leg, circle your left ankle in a clockwise direction three times. Then reverse the direction and circle your ankle counter-clockwise three times.

2) Bend your foot backwards and stretch your foot three times. Change sides and repeat.

CHAPTER TWELVE

STRETCHING

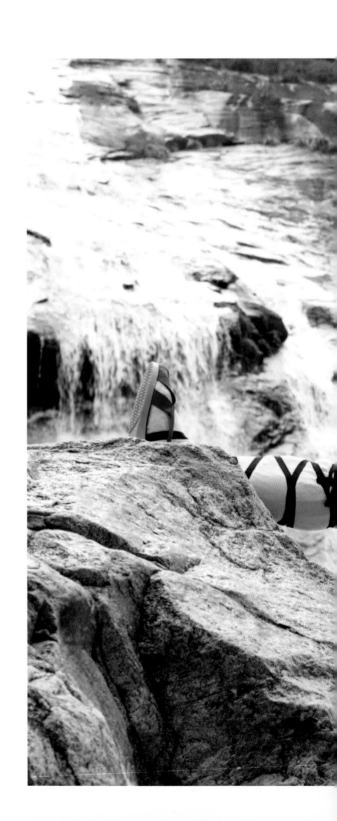

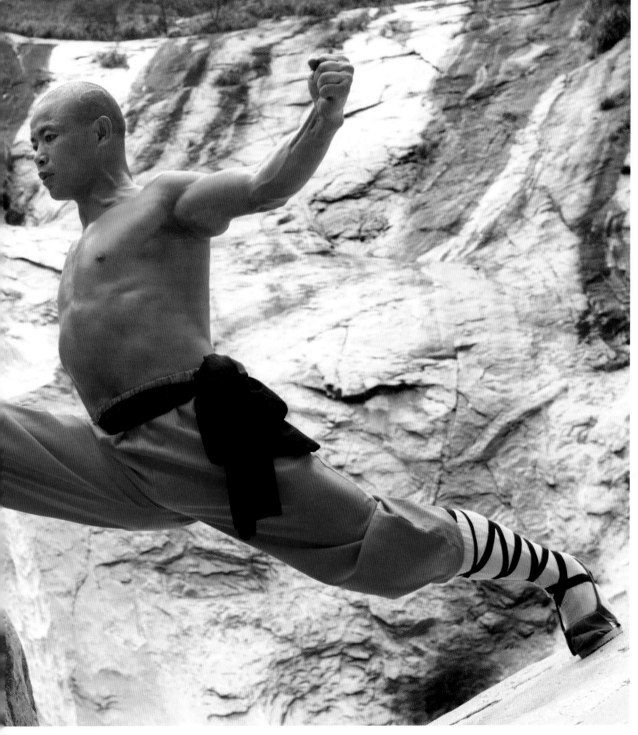

As I mentioned earlier on in the book, if you look at a picture of me stretching please don't feel discouraged. If you are as stiff as a board and your muscles are tight, after you have read the directions let your body move in the direction I am stretching. You will get as much benefit from your stretch as I do from mine and over time you will be surprised how flexible you will become. You don't need to be able to do the splits but you do need to have a certain degree of flexibility to prevent stiffness and to keep the body young. It is good to aim for the splits because it opens the hips and stretches the legs at the same time.

There should be no pain when you stretch but a gentle stretch that deepens as you breathe into it.

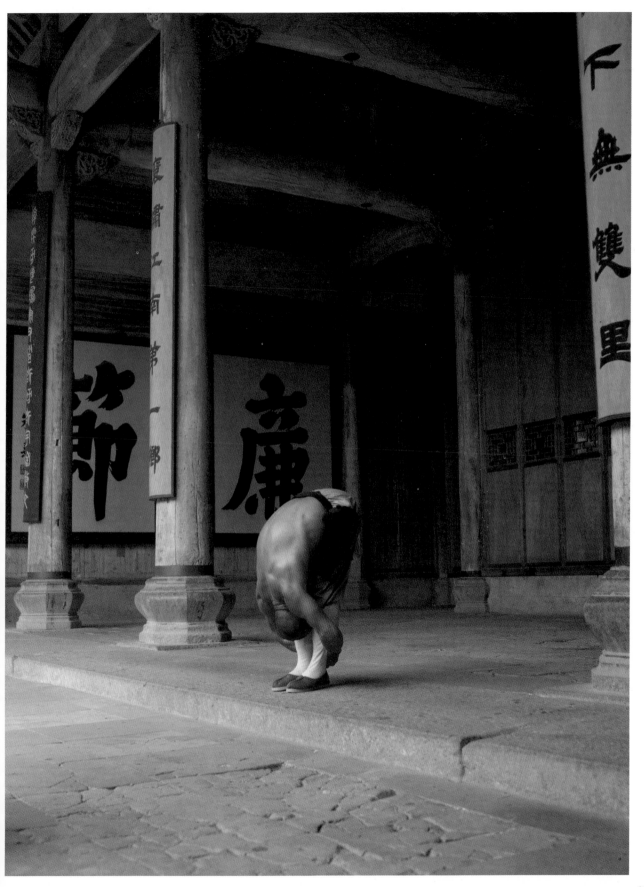

ARM STRETCHES
SHANG LA JIAN
UPPER STRETCH

ZUO LA JIAN
LEFT STRETCH

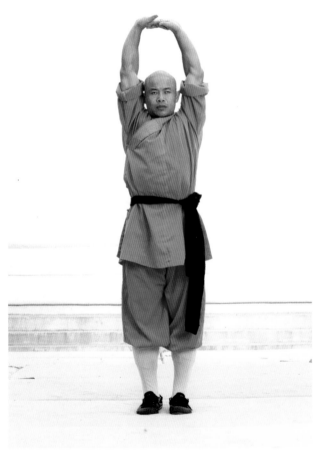

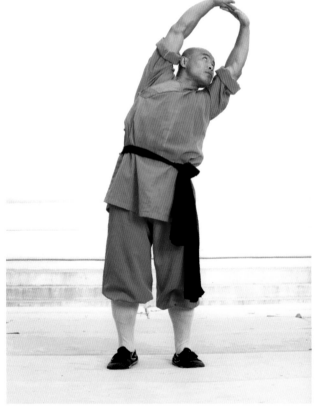

1) Interlace your hands and push your hands up to the sky as hard as you can. Keep your arms straight.
HOLD POSITION AND BREATHE x5

2) Bend your upper body to your left and stretch your arms as hard as you can. Keep your knees straight. Grab the floor with your feet.
HOLD POSITION AND BREATHE x5

YOU LA JIAN
RIGHT STRETCH

QIAN LA JIAN
FRONT STRETCH

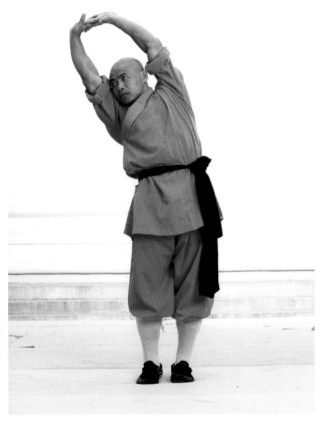

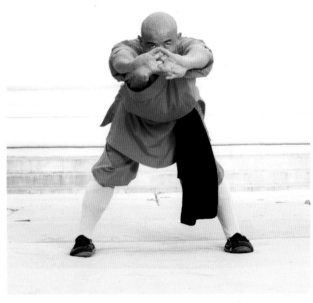

3) Bend your upper body to the right and stretch your arms as hard as you can.

HOLD POSITION AND BREATHE x5

Use your breath to increase the stretch. Keep your legs straight and your feet rooted to the ground. Your feet need to grab the floor, your back needs to be straight. Focus on your breathing and the direction of your hands. Move into...

4) Open your feet hip width apart, bend at the waist and stretch forward.

Drop your lower back and keep your knees straight. Hands push forward and eyes look forward.

HOLD POSITION AND BREATHE x5

BAO FO JIAO
HOLD BUDDHA'S FEET

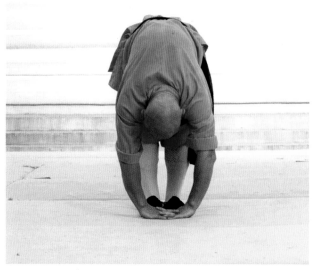

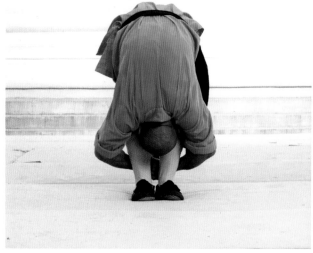

5) Bring your feet together.

Drop forward and try to touch the floor with your palms or fingers.
Keep your knees straight.

HOLD POSITION AND BREATHE x5

6) Place your hands behind your legs and interlace your fingers so your hands are holding your ankles. Place your head on your shin.

HOLD POSITION AND BREATHE x5

Don't push this stretch and always keep your legs straight. If you can't place your head on your shin don't worry, just keep your body dropped, your legs straight and breathe deeply in the stretch. Move into...

LEG STRETCHES
ZHENG YA TUI
FRONT LEG STRETCH

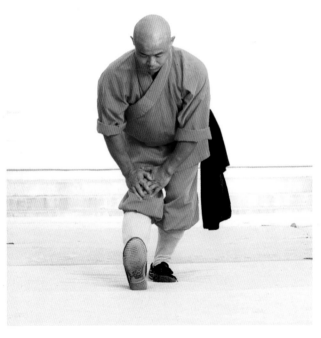
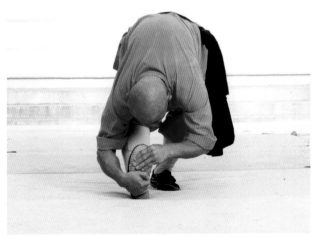

7) Bend your right knee and place your left leg straight out in front of you. Place both hands on your left knee. Lift your left foot onto the edge of the heel. Use your hands to keep your knee straight and stretch your body over your knee.
HOLD POSITION AND BREATHE x5

8) If you find this easy then clasp your front foot with both hands and try to place your head as far forward as possible. The aim is to touch your feet with your head.
HOLD POSITION AND BREATHE x5
Don't bend your back. Keep it straight.
Change sides and repeat. Go straight into…

CE YA TUI
SIDE STRETCH

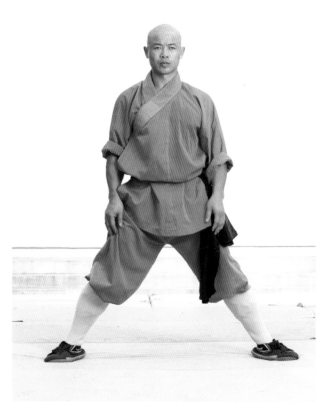

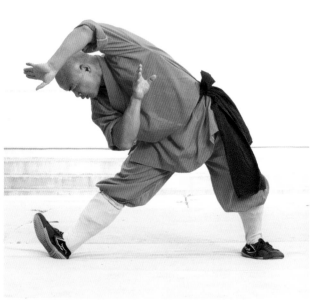

9) Bring your body up and place your legs hip width apart.

10) Raise your left arm over your head and place your right arm across your body. Stretch over to your right, bending your left leg and lifting your right foot so you are balanced on the ball of your foot. Keep your right leg straight.
HOLD POSITION AND BREATHE x5

11) If you find this stretch easy then lower your body and use both hands to grasp hold of your feet. Eyes look towards the left shoulder.

HOLD POSITION AND BREATHE x5

Change sides and repeat.

Don't collapse in your lower back but keep your body facing outwards. Feel a stretch through both sides of your body. It's better to stretch high and straight and only progress to movement 11) when you have the flexibility to do so.

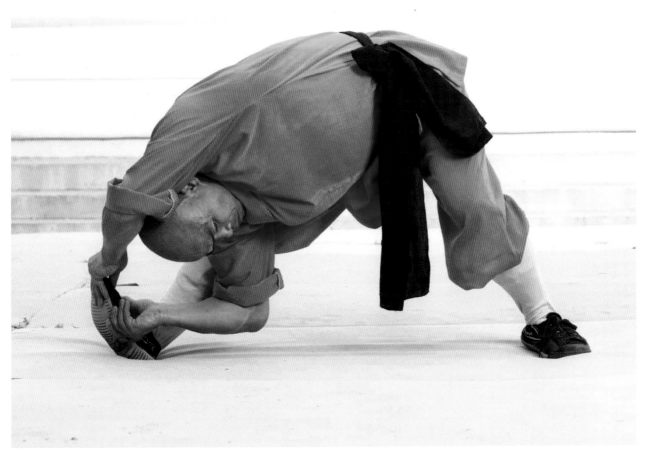

PU BU YA TUI

The next two stretching exercises use two stances from The Five Fundamental Stances, Pu Bu and Gong Bu. Learn the Five Fundamental Stances before doing these two stretches.

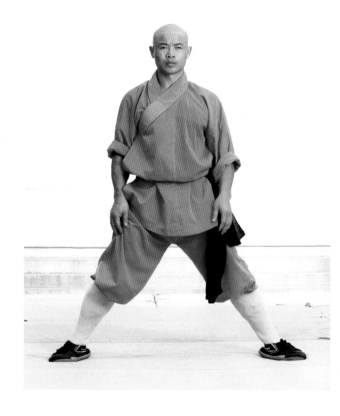

12) Stand straight. Feet hip-width apart.

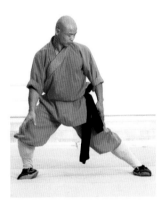 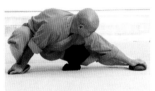 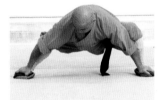 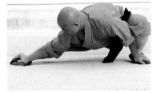

13) Bend your right knee, keeping your left leg straight.

14) Squat down into Pu Bu. Hold your right foot with your right hand and at the same time push out your knee with your elbow so it doesn't collapse inwards. Hold your left foot with your left hand.
HOLD POSITION AND BREATHE x5

15) Go into a very low Ma Bu, using both hands to hold both feet.

16) Change to the other side.
HOLD POSITION AND BREATHE x5
This exercise opens the hips. Don't worry if you cannot get low at first. The most important thing is to keep your back straight and your hips open, making sure your knees don't collapse inwards. If you can't hold your feet then you can put your hands on your knee.

GONG BU YA TUI

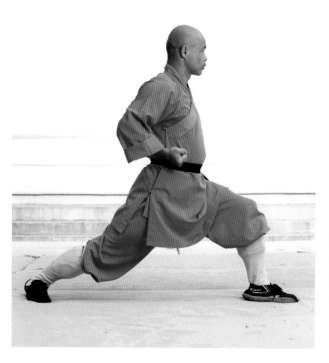

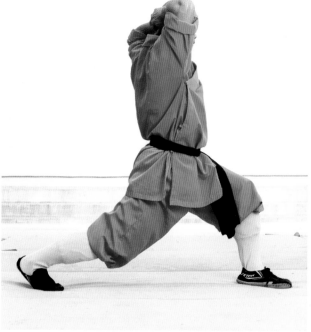

17) Stand up and turn to your left. Go into Gong Bu.

18) Interlace your fingers and place both hands on the back of your neck. Your front foot is flat, push the toes of your back foot and rise up onto the ball of your foot so that you feel a stretch in your calf muscle. Turn your body further to the left to increase the stretch in your leg.
HOLD POSITION AND BREATHE x3
Change sides and repeat.
This is a preparation for the splits.

SHU CHA
SPLITS

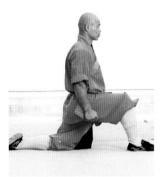 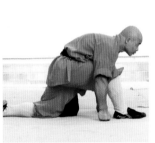 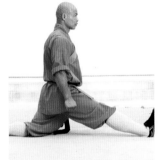 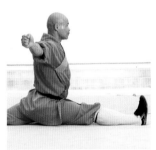

19) From Gong Bu bend your left knee onto the floor. Keep your feet flat. HOLD POSITION AND BREATHE x3

20) Place your fists on the floor and start to stretch out your back leg. HOLD POSITION AND BREATHE x3

21) Move your right leg forward by lifting your front foot up. Feel a stretch in your legs. HOLD POSITION AND BREATHE x3
If you find this easy then...

22) Lift your arms out to the side and move into the splits. HOLD POSITION AND BREATHE x3
Change sides and repeat.
Don't push this position. Practise a little every day and you will be surprised how closer you come to the floor.

HEN CHA
FORWARD SPLITS

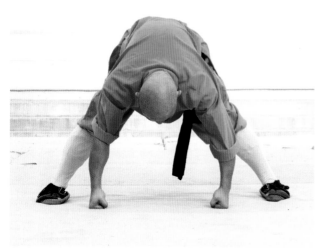

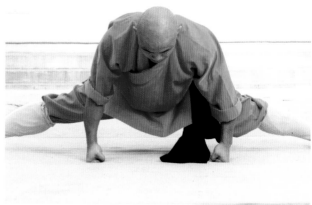

23) Move your body to the centre and touch the floor with your hands.

24) Stretch out your legs and slowly lower them to the floor.
HOLD POSITION AND BREATHE x5
If you find this easy then...

25) Place your legs flat on the floor. Bring your arms
out to the side. Keep your back straight.
HOLD POSITION AND BREATHE x5

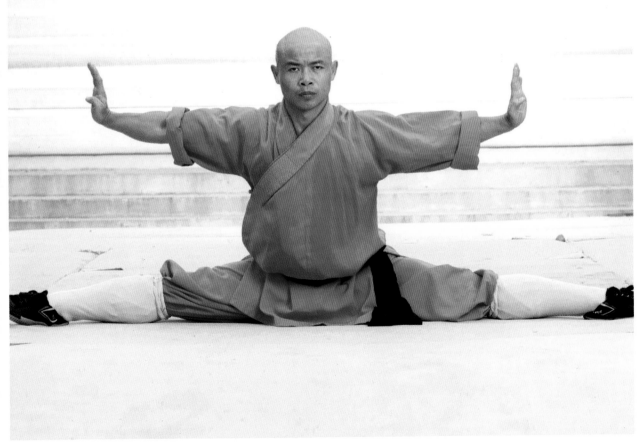

CHAPTER THIRTEEN

FIVE FUNDAMENTAL STANCES

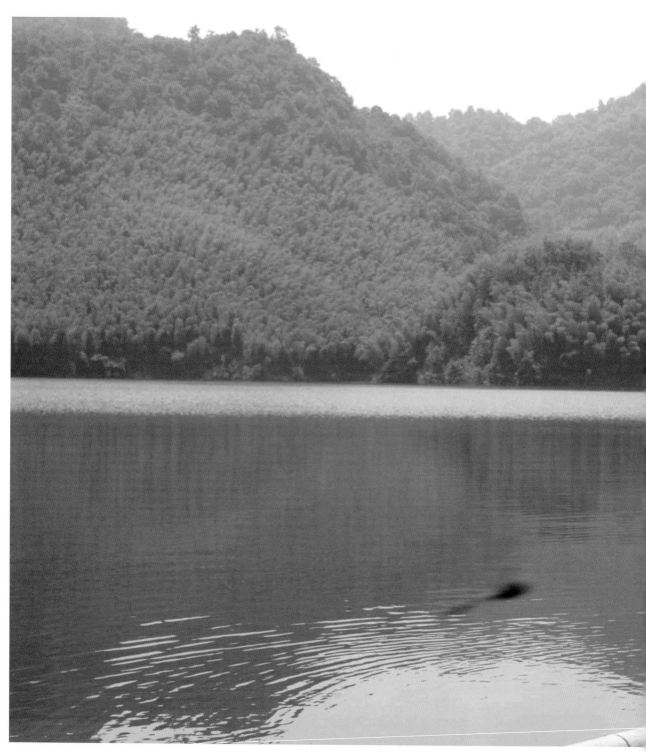

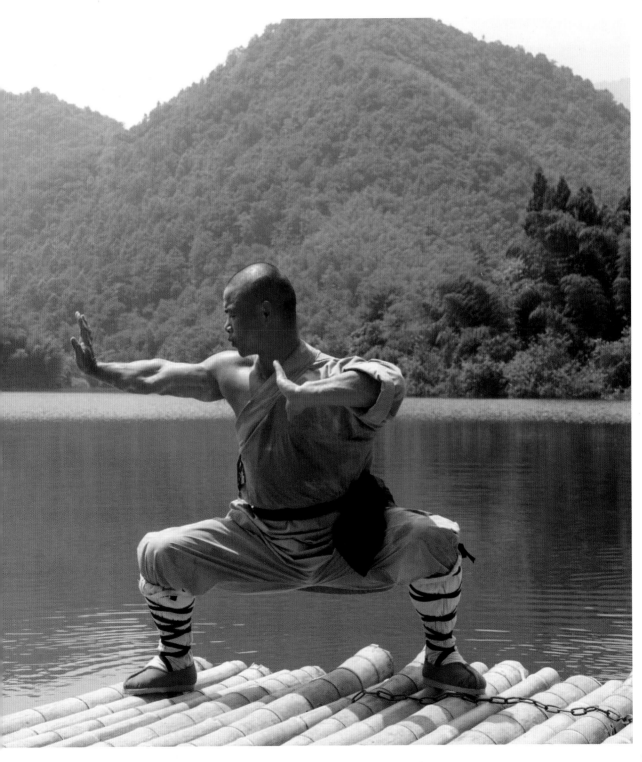

THE FIVE FUNDAMENTAL STANCES:

Are the keys to learning the Shaolin forms
Strengthen your legs
Build your co-ordination and balance

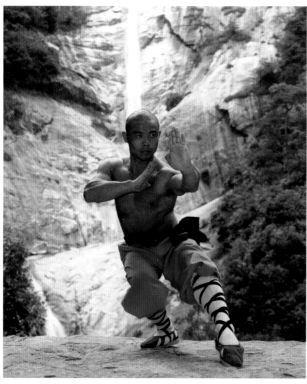

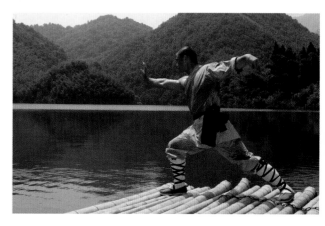

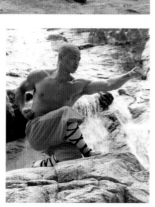

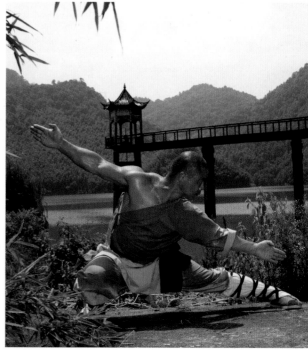

If you have seen the Shaolin monks do a performance, I'm sure you will agree they look beautiful. These five stances form the foundation of all Shaolin forms. In order to learn any form whether it is a Qigong form or a Kung Fu form you must learn the Five Fundamental Stances first. All Shaolin forms consist of these stances, which are then linked together with punches, jumps, kicks and blocks.

Older people or people with less flexibility should do the stances much higher than me. I do low stances, and all seasoned martial artists should do the same but you will get as much benefit if your stance is high. Listen to your body and work with it.

When you practise the five stances the most important thing is to feel stable in the stance. If you are not stable, this means that when you move on to practise forms your form will not be stable either. When you first begin it is a good idea to check your stance in the mirror. Is your back straight? Is your behind tucked in? Are you grabbing the floor with your feet? Are your eyes focused? Remember - we use every part of our body when we practise Shaolin including our eyes and our mind.

It will take about three months to build the strength of your legs. In some stances, we build up both legs and in other stances we build up one leg or a combination of the two, with different percentages of weight balanced on different sides. The best way to practise the stances is by staying in each stance for a few minutes and then moving on. Keep the stance as low as you can and, as you get tired, heighten the stance. You can try the opposite way too.

The stances don't just help you to practise your forms, they also build up your will power. If you stay in Ma Bu for two minutes and your legs start to shake, your body wants to stand up and you have to use the power of your mind to push yourself to stay a little longer. We call this static stamina because although there is no movement there is effort. When you have finished your stance work, it is a good idea to give your body a shake out or practise some traditional punches and kicks to loosen up any stiffness in the legs. Make sure the knee - foot alignment is correct. There should be no pain in the knee. If there is then you are doing something incorrectly and need to stop.

MA BU
HORSE STANCE

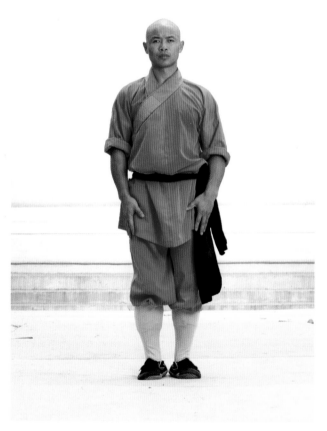

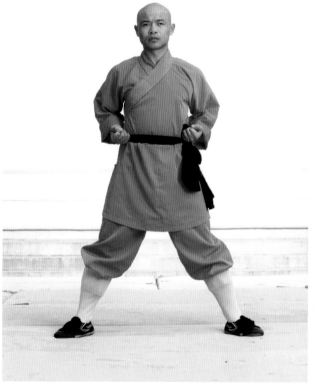

1) Stand straight.

2) Step your left leg out to the side so your feet are wider than the shoulders. At the same time make fists with your hands and draw them into the waist.

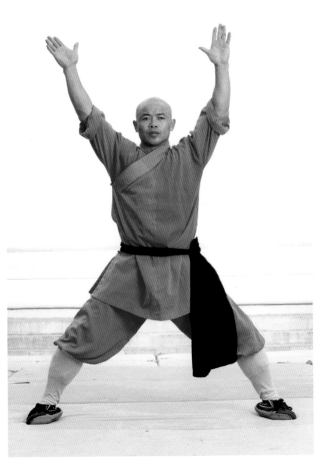

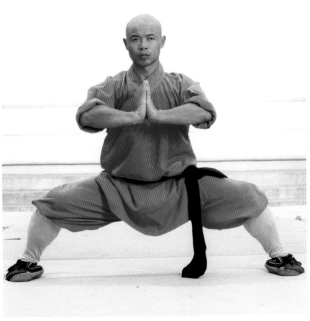

3) 4) Lift both hands above your head and bring them down into a prayer position in front of your chest. At the same time squat down into Ma Bu.

REMAIN HERE FOR SIX BREATHS.

Eyes look forward. Feet grab the floor. Push your knees out a little and don't let them collapse. Tuck your behind in slightly. Elbows go up and wrists go down. Open your chest. Keep your centre of gravity in the middle.

GONG BU

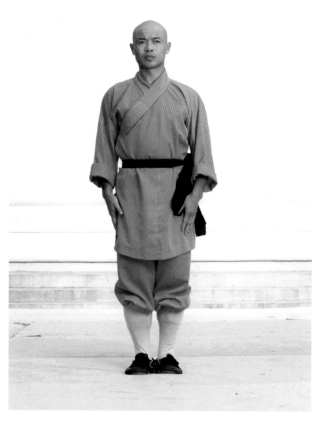

1) Stand straight.

2) Draw your fists to your waist and open your chest. Turn your head to look to the left.

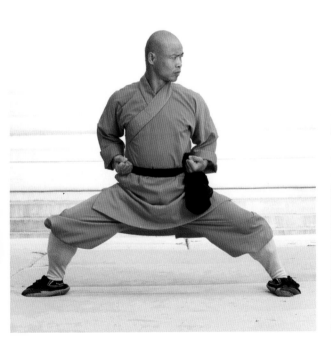

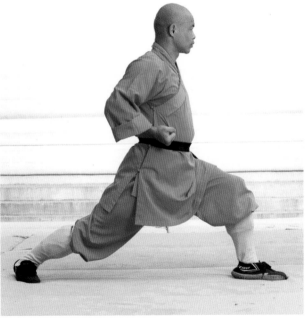

3) Step your left leg out to the side and squat into horse stance.

4) Turn both legs and bend your left leg as much as you can, keeping your right leg straight. Turn your body to face the left.
REMAIN HERE FOR SIX BREATHS.
REPEAT ON THE OTHER SIDE.
Your right foot should be slightly turned in, it shouldn't be completely straight and needs to be in line with your left foot.

PU BU

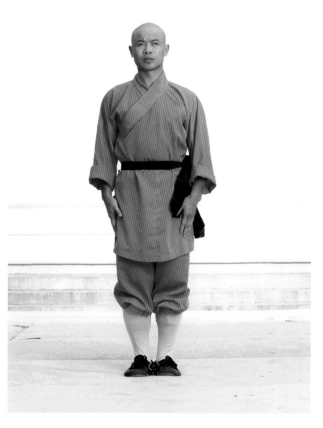

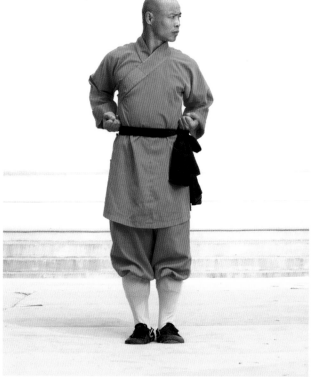

1) Stand straight.

2) Draw your fists to your waist and open your chest. Turn your head to look to the left.

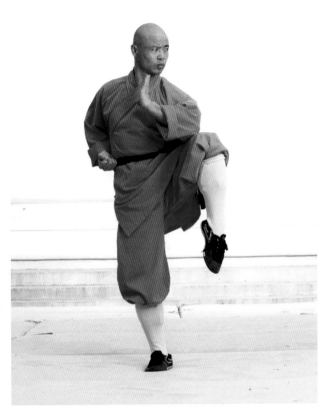

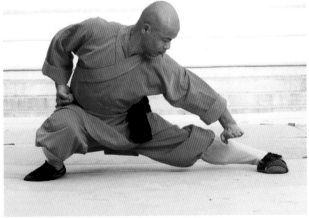

3) Raise your left knee and bring your left hand to your chest.

4) Bend your right knee and squat down until your left leg is straight on the floor. Turn your palm outwards and try to get your palm as close to the left foot as possible.
REMAIN HERE FOR SIX BREATHS.
REPEAT ON THE OTHER SIDE.
More than 70% of gravity is on your right leg. If you can't place your hand on your foot then place it on your knee or thigh.

XIE BU

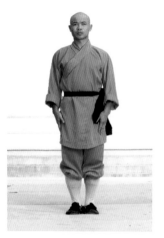 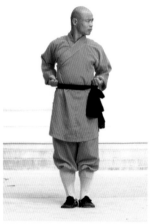 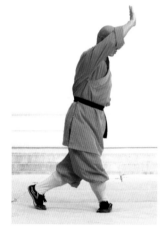 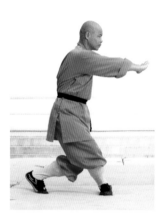

1) Stand straight.

2) Draw your fists to your waist and open your chest. Turn your head to look to the left.

3) Step your left leg behind your right leg. Raise your right hand and bring it across your head as if you are blocking something.

4) 5) Squat down onto your left leg. At the same time your right palm changes into a fist and draws back into your waist.

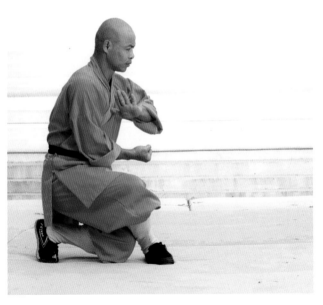 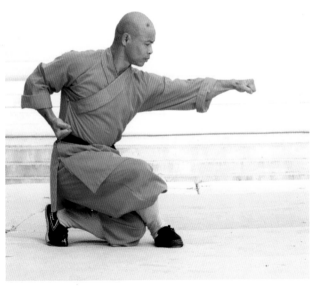

6) Punch out straight with your left hand.
REMAIN HERE FOR SIX BREATHS.
REPEAT ON THE OTHER SIDE.

XUE BU

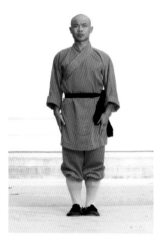 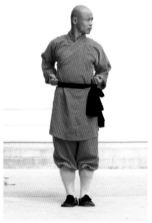 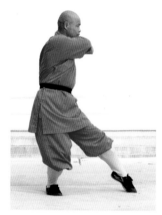 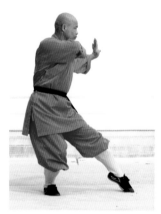

1) Stand straight.

2) Draw your fists to your waist and open your chest. Turn your head to look to the left.

3) 4) Step your left leg out a little to the side. Turn your body and draw half a circle with both hands – your left hand draws a circle in front of your chest, your right hand draws a bigger circle outside your body.

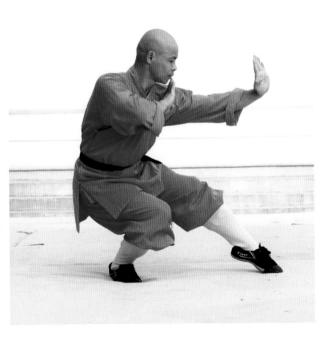

Apart from Ma Bu, repeat the movements on the opposite side. If your left leg is in front it's called "Zuo Gong Bu". If your right leg is in front it is called, "You Gong Bu". You can also link these five stances together.
I show you how to do this in my second book: Instant Fitness: The Shaolin Kungfu Workout.

5) Bend both knees.
REMAIN HERE FOR SIX BREATHS.
REPEAT ON THE OTHER SIDE.
95% of the weight should be on your back leg. Check by lifting your left leg.

CHAPTER FOURTEEN

HOW TO GET THE MOST FROM YOUR QIGONG WORKOUT

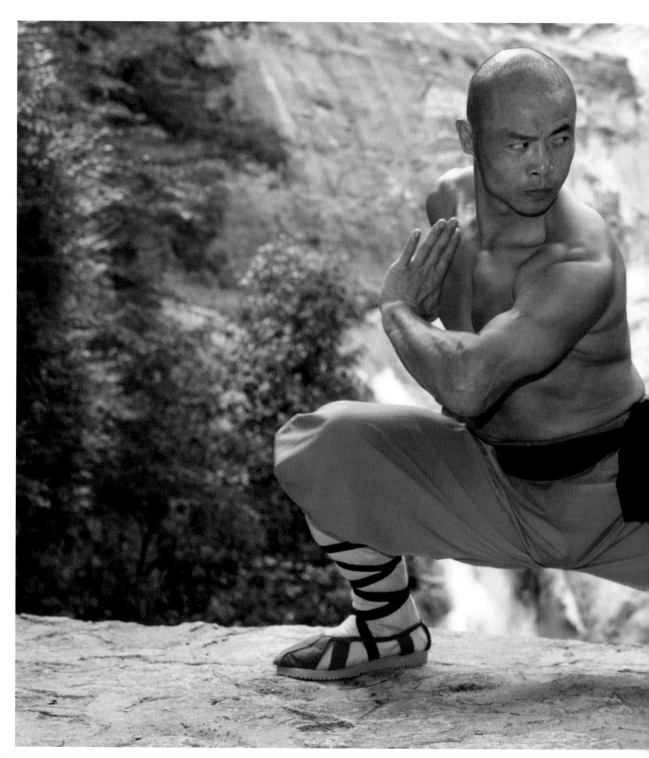

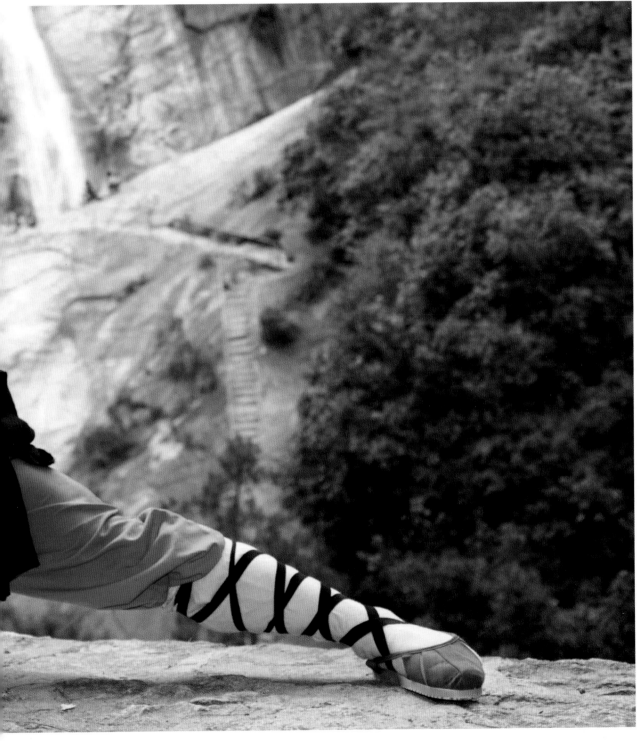

DYNAMIC STRETCH

When we hold the Qigong postures we use a dynamic stretch to activate the energy so we are not just holding the movement but are also opening up our body. Qi cannot flow through a tense muscle nor can it flow through a limp wrist. We use minimum effort for maximum stretch. When you have completed the form, your arms and legs should feel tired. If they don't it means that you are not using enough power. When you make your arms straight you need to make your wrist straight, and you need to use your mind to tell your body to use power. This power shouldn't be tense but gentle. True relaxation is often compared to water; soft, supple, alive and powerful.

CIRCLE THE HANDS

The direction of the hands is important. Look at the first movement; we don't just raise our hands to make a small ball but we circle them up and out. These hand movements may seem small but they need to be correct as this helps with the flow of energy.

HOW TO LEARN

You need to have learnt the Five Fundamental Stances and Complete Qigong Breathing before beginning to learn this form. This will make it easier to learn the form and your practice will be more effective. Start by reading through Tuo Tian Shi – Push The Sky, and go over it a few times. Once you have memorized it without much prompting from the book you can then progress to the next section.

THE QIGONG WORKOUT

For a good Qigong workout I recommend you work through the whole workout in this book including the warm up, stretching and massage. Practise The Eight Treasures form with a break of three breaths in between, and hold each movement for the correct amount of breaths as stated next to the picture. Once you know the form you can break it down and practise just one or two of the sections. Alternatively, you can hold the movements that are usually held for three breaths for one.

Even a few minutes of Qigong practice will make you feel more energised. If you're pushed for time, start with five minutes a day. Five minutes a day counts. By the end of the year it amounts to 1825 minutes towards a healthier you.

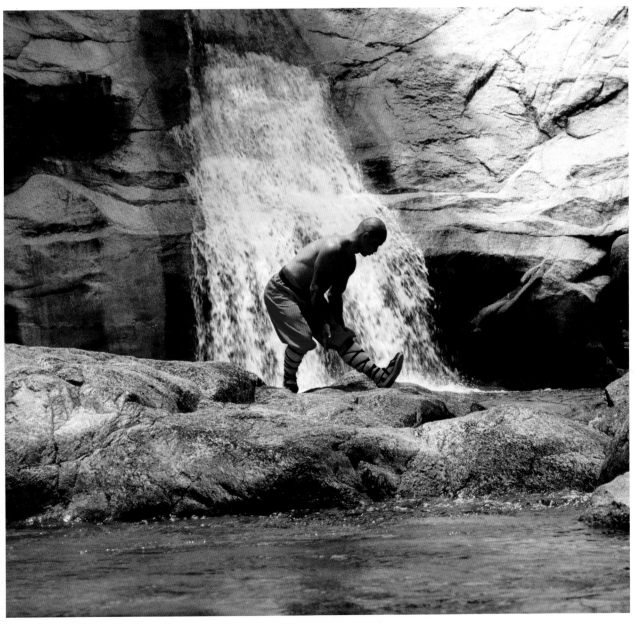

CHAPTER FIFTEEN

THE COMPLETE
EIGHT TREASURES FORM

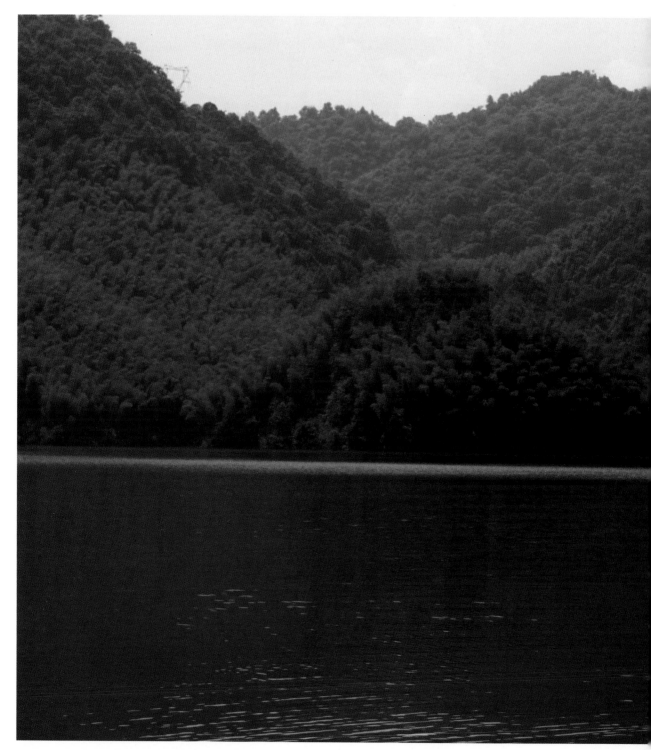

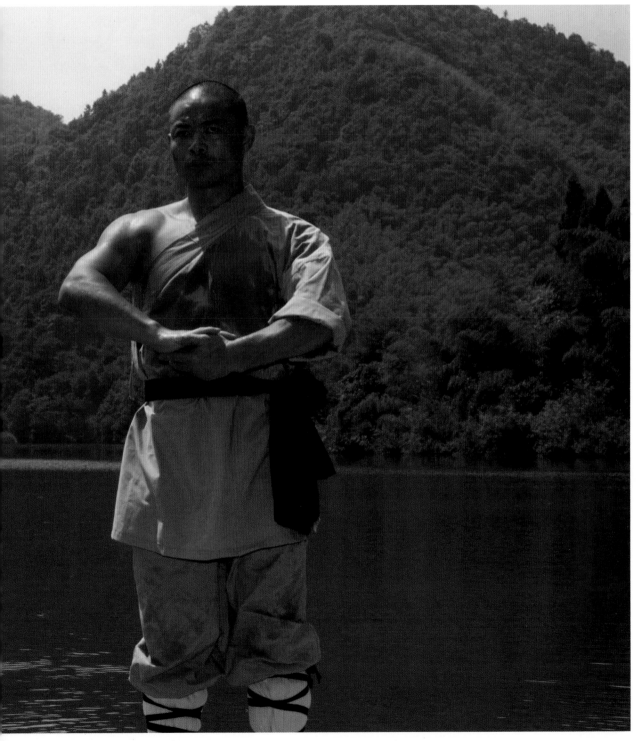

1ST MOVEMENT

In this sequence you need to make sure that your arm is straight by pushing out with your hands.

TUO TIAN SHI
PUSH THE SKY

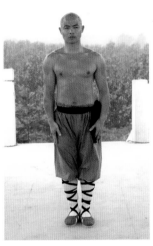
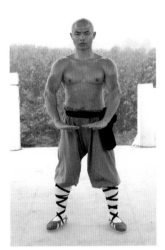
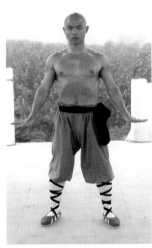
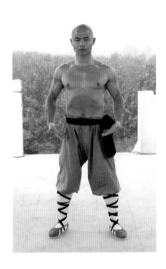

1) Stand in a neutral position with both arms at your side.
REMAIN HERE FOR THREE BREATHS.

2) Step your left foot out to the side, at the same time bring your arms in front of your body and turn your hands so your palms face the ground.

3) Inhale. Keep turning your hands and bring them out to the side.

4) Continue to turn your hands and bring them to the front of your body.

TUO TIAN SHI
PUSH THE SKY

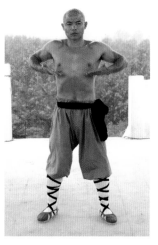 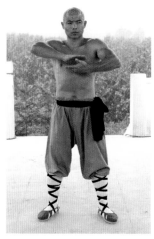 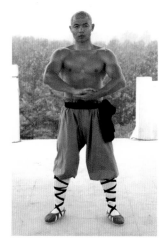 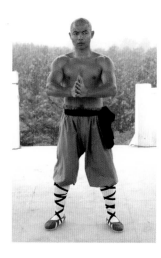

5) Draw them up to your chest and push your elbows back as far as they will go. Feel your chest expand.

6a 6b) Exhale. Place your right hand on top of your left hand as if your hands are holding one small ball and your elbows are holding a bigger ball. Look straight in front of you.

REMAIN HERE FOR THREE BREATHS.

Make sure your shoulders are dropped and relaxed. Slightly press your shoulders down and open your chest so that you feel an internal stretch from the shoulders all the way down the arms into your fingers.

7) Inhale. Turn your right hand and place it level with your left hand, your fingers pointing straight out in front of you.

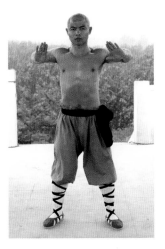 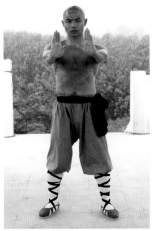 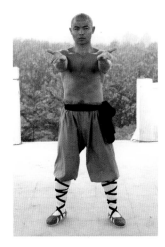 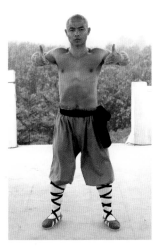

8) Bring your palms back to your chest and push your elbows back as far as they will go. Feel your chest expand.

9) Exhale. Turn your hands and use the side of your hands to push out in front of you. Look at your hands. Bend your wrists back to engage the stretch.

10) Inhale. Turn your palms so they are facing the sky.

11) Bring your palms back to your chest and push your elbows back as far as they will go. Feel your chest expand.

TUO TIAN SHI
PUSH THE SKY

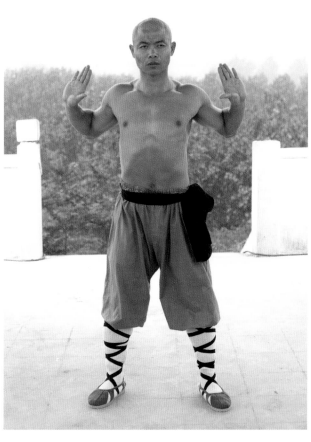

12) Exhale. Turn your palms.

13) Push both arms out to the side. Bend your wrists back to engage the stretch. Eyes look at your left hand. REMAIN HERE FOR THREE BREATHS.

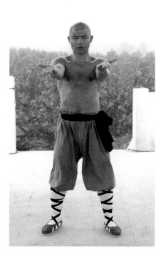 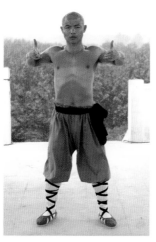 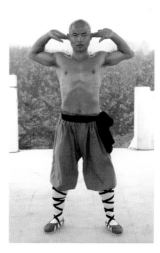 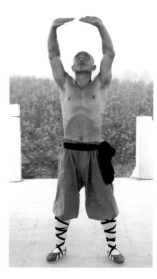

14) Inhale. Circle your arms back to your chest, palms facing the sky.

15) Bring your palms back to your chest and push your elbows back as far as they will go. Feel your chest expand.

16) 17) Exhale. Stretch your hands over your head and push your palms up to the sky as if you are trying to push the sky away from you. Bend your wrists back to engage the stretch. Eyes look upwards.

REMAIN HERE FOR THREE BREATHS.

TUO TIAN SHI
PUSH THE SKY

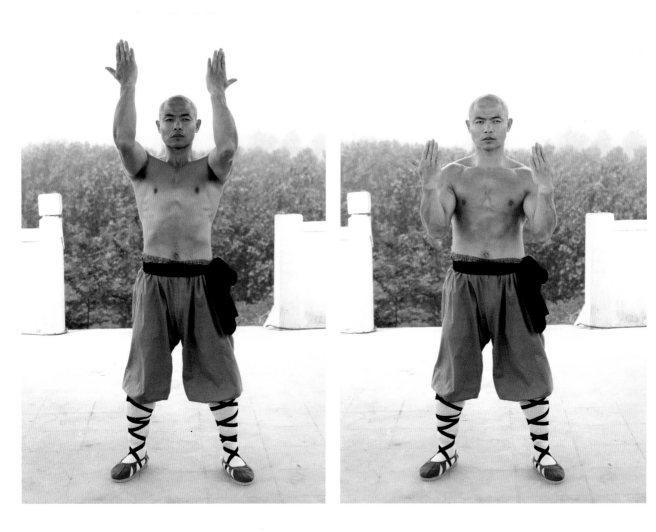

18) 19) Inhale. Slowly lower your arms and turn your palms so that they face your body.

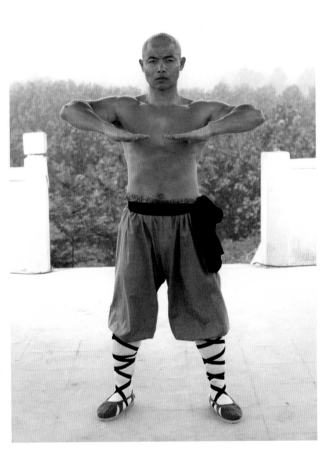

20) Exhale. Flatten your palms and slowly push your arms down.

21) Bring both feet together.
REMAIN HERE FOR THREE BREATHS.

2ND MOVEMENT

In this sequence the most important thing is to be stable. We practice two of the Five Fundamental Stances, Ma Bu and Gong Bu. Remember to practise these stances as high or as low as is within your comfort level. Our arms make the shape of firing an arrow from a bow.

KAI GONG SHI
BOW AND ARROW

START FROM NEUTRAL POSITION

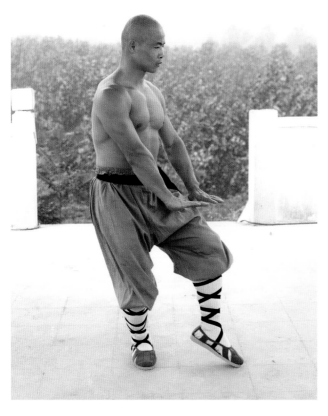

1) Inhale. Turn to the left. Move the weight onto your right leg, slightly bend your knee and lift up onto the ball of your left foot. Place your palms flat on either side of your knee.

2) Raise your left knee and at the same time turn your palms to face the sky.

KAI GONG SHI
BOW AND ARROW

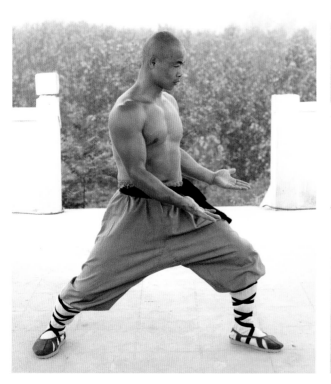

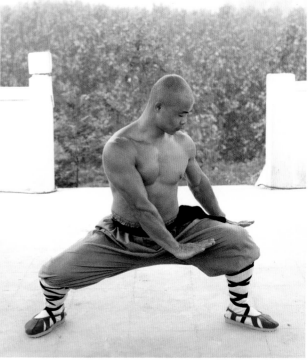

3) Place your foot on the floor hip-width apart.

4) Exhale. Squat and push both hands down on either side of your knee. Palms facing the floor.
70% of the weight is on your left side.

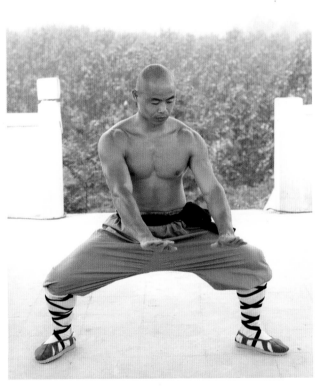 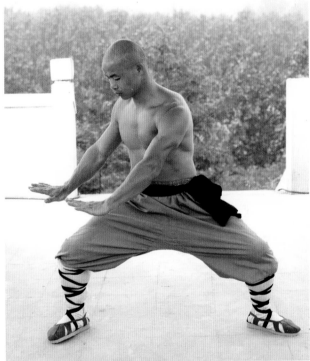

5) 6) Inhale. Turn your arms and your body to the centre,
then over to your right side.

Now you're going to repeat exactly what you did on the other side.

KAI GONG SHI
BOW AND ARROW

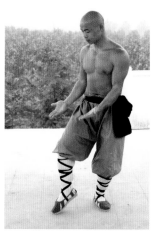 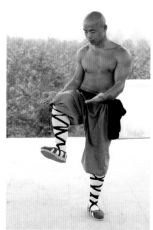 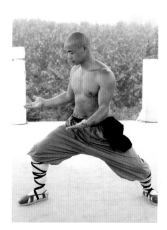 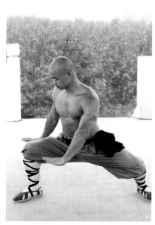

7) Move your weight onto your back leg and lift up your right foot. Place your palms on either side of your knee. Palms facing the sky.

8) Raise your right knee.

9) Drop your foot onto the floor, hip-width apart.

10) Exhale. Squat and push both hands down on either side of your knee. Palms facing the floor.
70% of the weight is on your right side.

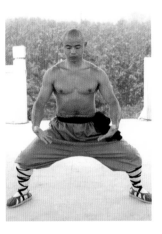 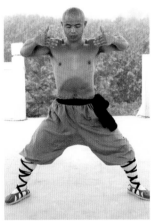 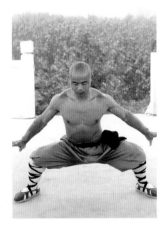 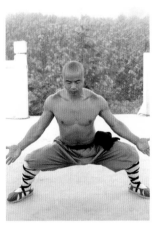

11) Inhale. Turn your body to the centre and go into Ma Bu. At the same time make a circle with your arms, palms facing the sky.

12) Raise your arms to your chest and come up a little higher in Ma Bu.

13) Exhale. Squat and push your palms down on either side of your knees.

14) Inhale. Turn your palms.

KAI GONG SHI
BOW AND ARROW

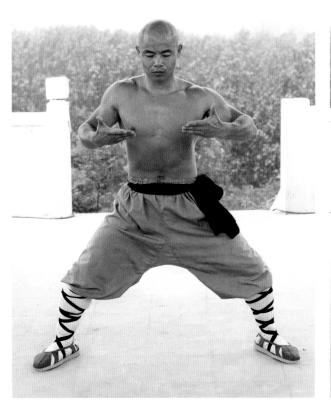

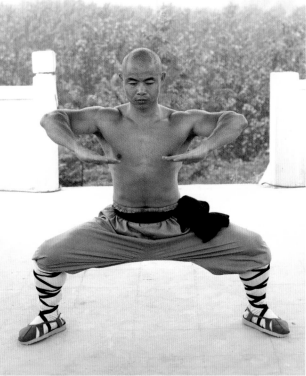

15) Come up a little higher in Ma Bu and raise your arms to your chest. Palms facing the sky.

16) Exhale. Push your palms down in the middle of your body and squat into Ma Bu.
Make sure your centre of gravity is in the middle.

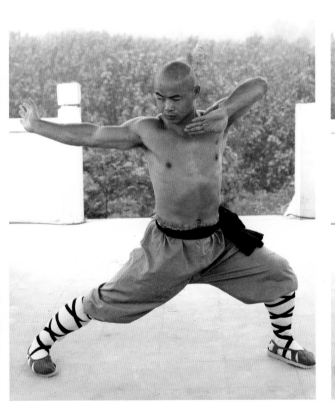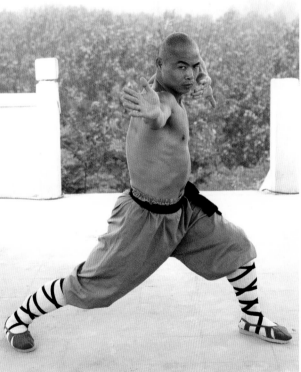

17) Inhale. Turn your left foot and go into a high Pu Bu. Bend your left elbow and bring your hand below your chin, taking your right hand out to the side.

18) Slowly move your body and your right arm towards the left.

KAI GONG SHI
BOW AND ARROW

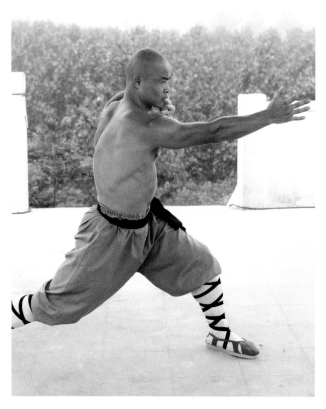

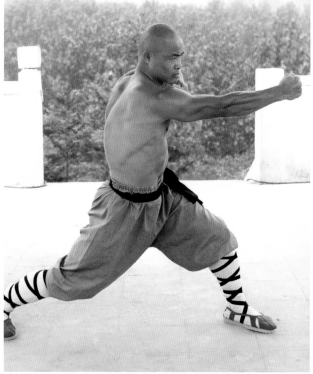

19) Keep moving your body and your right arm until it is all the way over to your left.

20) Make a fist with your right hand as if you are grabbing hold of something and at the same time flatten the palm of your left hand.

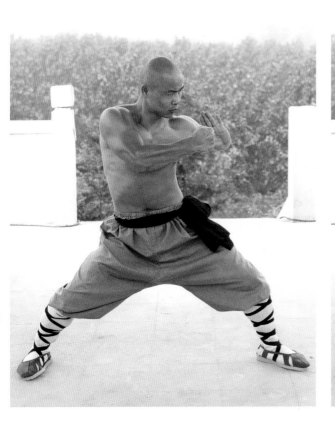

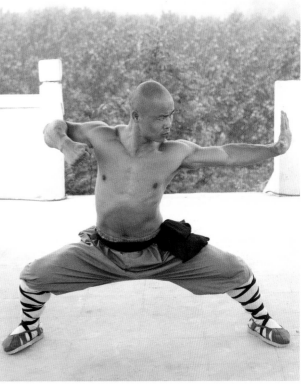

21) Exhale. Draw your right arm back as if you are firing an arrow from a bow. At the same time begin to push your left hand out to the side.

22) Push your left hand out to the side and squat into Ma Bu. Eyes look to your left. Make sure your arms and shoulders are even and straight.
REMAIN HERE FOR THREE BREATHS.

KAI GONG SHI
BOW AND ARROW

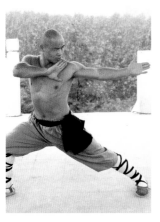 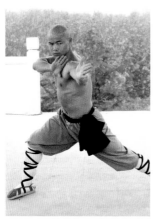 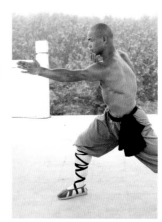 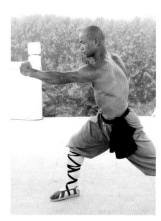

23) - 25) Inhale. Un-clasp your fist and turn your arm and upper body over to your right.

26) Make a fist with your left hand as if you are grabbing hold of something and at the same time flatten the palm of your right hand.

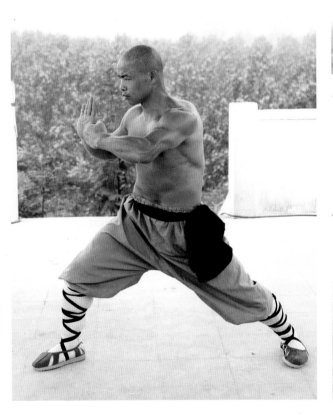 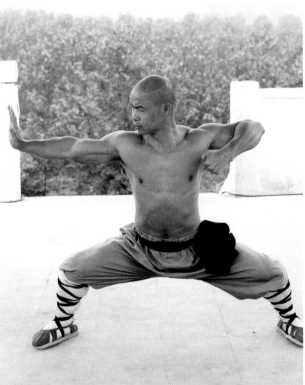

27) Exhale. Draw your left arm back as if you are firing an arrow from a bow. At the same time push your right hand out to the side.

28) Squat into Ma Bu. Eyes look to your right. REMAIN HERE FOR THREE BREATHS.

KAI GONG SHI
BOW AND ARROW

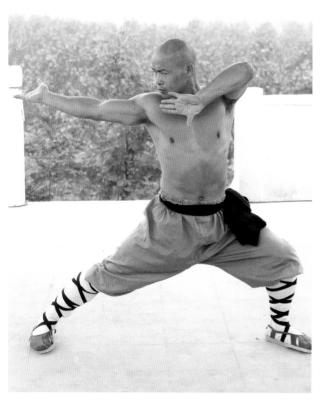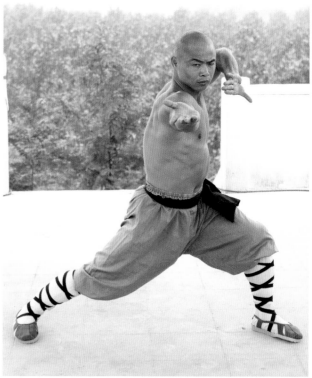

29) 30) Un-clasp your fist and turn your arm and upper body to the centre.

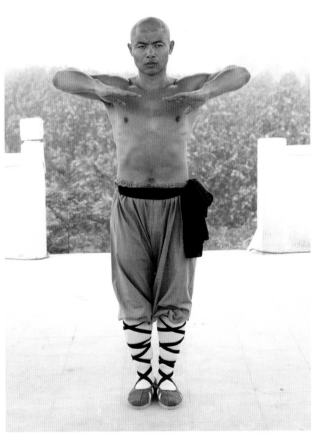 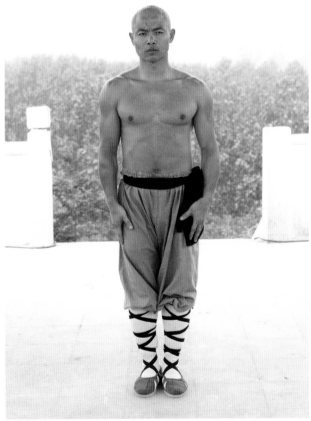

31) Step your right foot in so your feet are hip width apart. At the same time bend your elbows and turn your palms to face the ground. Exhale. Push down with your palms.

32) Close your feet and drop your arms. REMAIN HERE FOR THREE BREATHS.

3RD MOVEMENT

In this sequence when you push your hands you need to turn your wrist and then push. It is the same with your body; only turn your body, not your legs.

This sequence is called Dan Jue Shi, which means one hand plucking the stars. Another name is Ba Dao Shi. The old warriors always carried their sword behind their back, and the movement is similar to them taking their sword out of its holster. This sequence looks easy to do, but remember to use energy when you hold your arms up and down. Always activate the stretch and grab the floor with your feet.

DAN JUE SHI
ONE HAND PLUCKING THE STARS

START FROM NEUTRAL POSITION

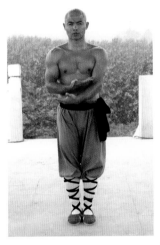 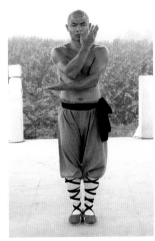

1) Inhale. Cross your arms in front of your body. Right arm on top.

2) 3) Bring your right palm across your face and your left palm under your elbow. Keep turning your wrist until your palm is across your face and your left arm around your body.

DAN JUE SHI
ONE HAND PLUCKING THE STARS

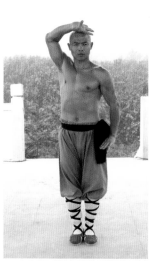
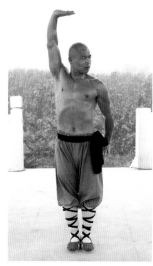
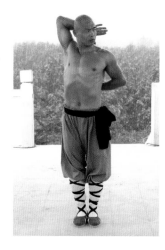
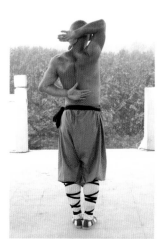

4) 5) Exhale. Your right arm pushes the sky, your left arm pushes the ground. At the same time turn your head to look over to your left. Bend your wrists to engage the stretch.

REMAIN HERE FOR THREE BREATHS.
Eyes look over to your left.
Keep your shoulders dropped.

6) Inhale. Bend both elbows and bring your left arm behind your back and place your palm on your left kidney. Place your right arm behind your head. Keep your palm and fingers straight.
To make sure your hand is in the right position, bend it and touch your ear. If you can touch your ear then it is in the right place.

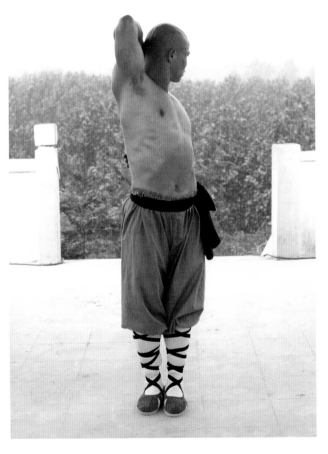

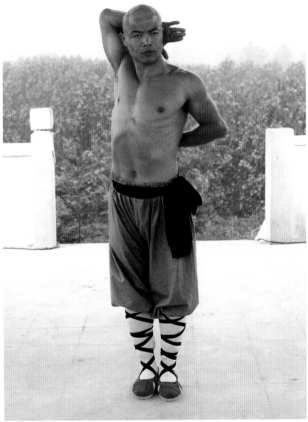

7) Exhale. Turn from your waist to your left until you can't turn anymore.

Don't move your legs. Check your knees are straight. Eyes follow your left shoulder.

8) Come back to the centre. Inhale.
REPEAT STEPS 6 -7 x3

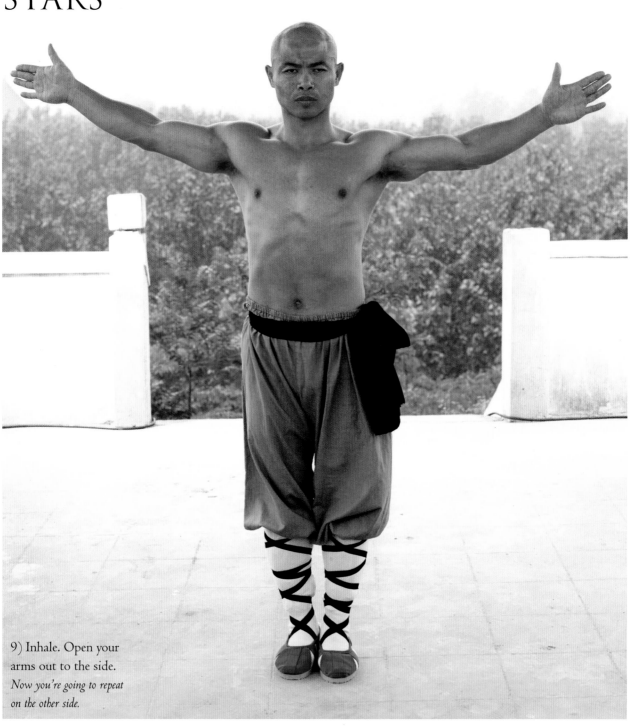

DAN JUE SHI
ONE HAND PLUCKING THE STARS

9) Inhale. Open your arms out to the side. *Now you're going to repeat on the other side.*

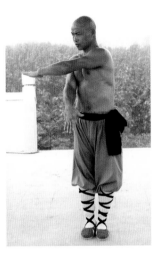 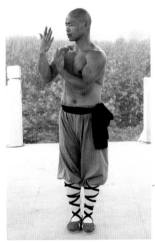 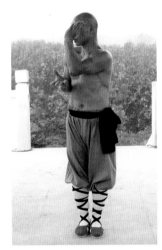 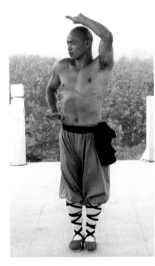

10) Cross your arms in front of your body. Your left arm on top, your right arm below.

11) 12) Bring your left palm across your face and your right hand down to your waist. Keep raising your left arm and lowering your right arm, turn your left palm outwards.

13) Exhale. Push your left arm towards the sky and your right arm downwards.

DAN JUE SHI
ONE HAND PLUCKING THE STARS

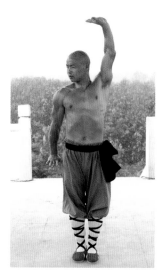 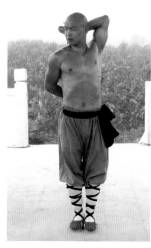 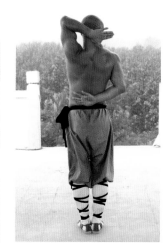 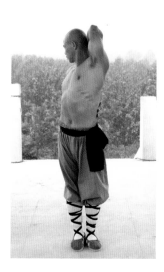

14) Bend your wrists to engage the stretch. REMAIN HERE FOR THREE BREATHS.

15) Inhale. Bend both elbows and bring your left arm behind your back and place your right palm on your right kidney. Place your left arm behind your head. Keep your palm and fingers straight.

16) Exhale. Turn from your waist to your right until you can't turn anymore.

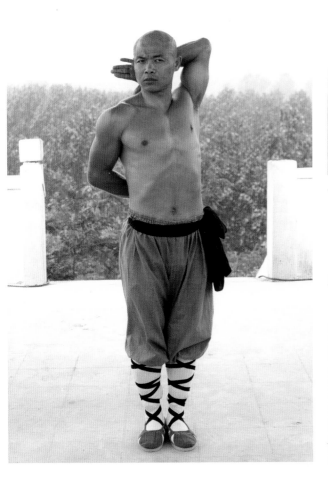

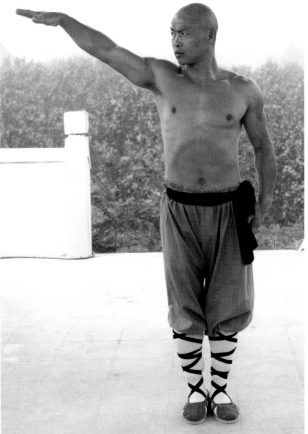

17) Come back to the centre. Inhale.
REPEAT STEPS 15 - 16 x3

18) Inhale. Drop your left hand down and move your right hand up.

DAN JUE SHI
ONE HAND PLUCKING THE STARS

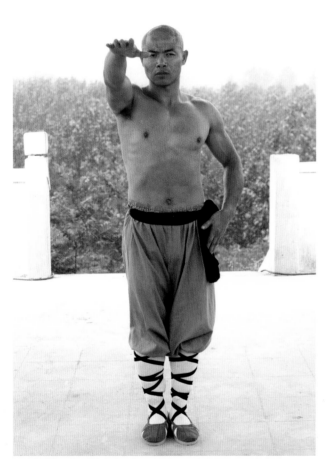

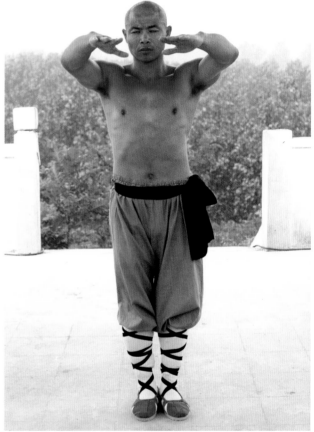

19) Move your right hand to the front of your body.

20) 21) Exhale. Bring your left arm up to the front of your body and push your arms down the front of your body.

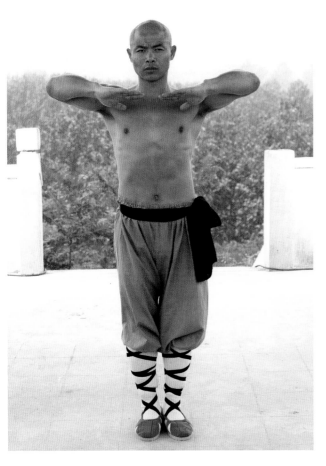 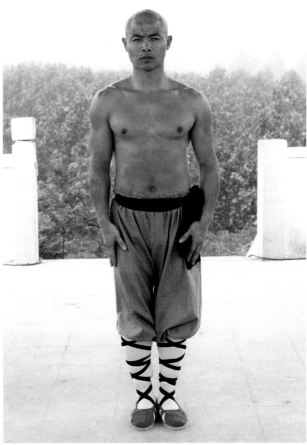

22) Stand straight.
HOLD POSITION AND BREATHE x3

4TH MOVEMENT

In this sequence you focus on the movement of the body. When you "take your shoes off" you move your upper body all the time. When you go to the second part then you move your head but you use your hips to move your head rather than your upper body. In China we say, "You move your head, you turn your tail, you cool your body down." This balances Yin and Yang.

The first part of this sequence is as if we are reaching to our feet to take our shoes off.

The second part is called Tou Sue Shi - Move your head. But you can call all of this sequence either "Yao Tou Shi" or "Tou Sue Shi".

YAO TOU SHI
TAKE YOUR SHOES OFF

START FROM NEUTRAL POSITION

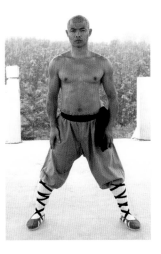 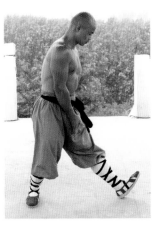 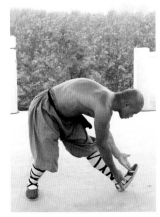 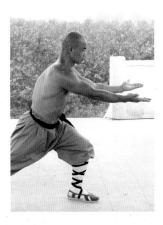

1) Step your left foot out to the side.

2) Inhale. Turn to your left and tip your left foot back onto the edge of the heel of your foot. Palms on either side of your leg.

3) Slightly bend your back leg and scoop your body down, reaching for your left foot as if you are trying to take your shoes off.

4) Continue the movement by dropping your feet down so you are in Gong Bu. Stretch your arms out in front of you.

YAO TOU SHI
TAKE YOUR SHOES OFF

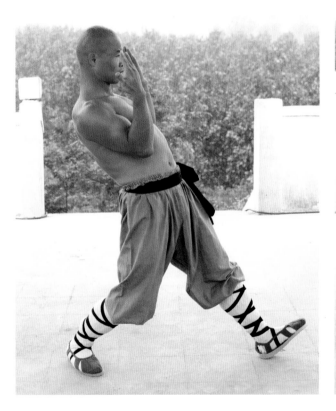

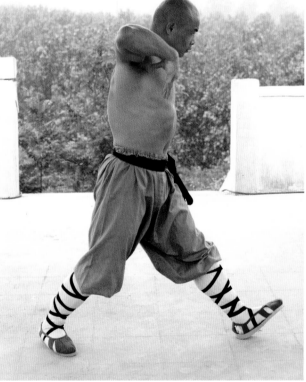

5) Bring your palms to your face, slightly bend your right knee and at the same time tip back a little onto your back foot so your front foot is on the edge of your heel.

6) Exhale. Turn your palms and move your body forward.

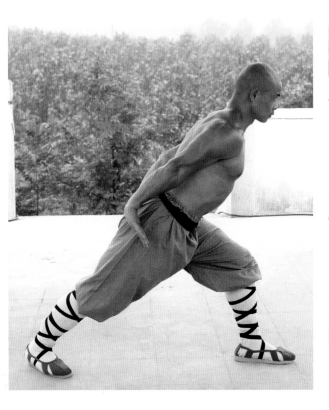 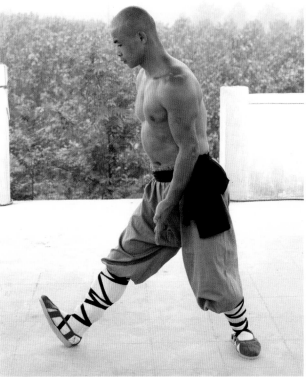

7) Go into Gong Bu. Push your palms down and push your head. Slightly tip your body over your left leg but make sure your back is straight.
REMAIN HERE FOR THREE BREATHS.
Now you're going to repeat on the other side.

8) Inhale. Turn to the right and tip your right foot onto the edge of your heel.

YAO TOU SHI
TAKE YOUR SHOES OFF

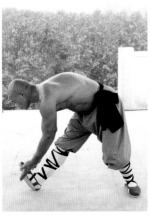
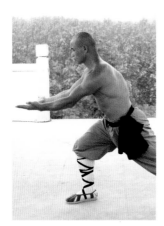
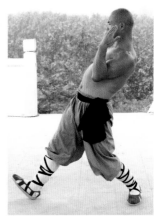
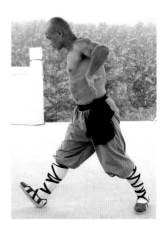

9) Slightly bend your back leg and scoop your body down, reaching for your right foot as if you are trying to take your shoes off.

10) Continue the movement by dropping your feet down so you are in Gong Bu and stretching your arms out in front of you.

11) Bring your palms to your face, slightly bend your left knee and at the same time tip back a little onto your back foot so your front foot is on the edge of the heel.

12) Exhale. Turn your palms and move your body forward.

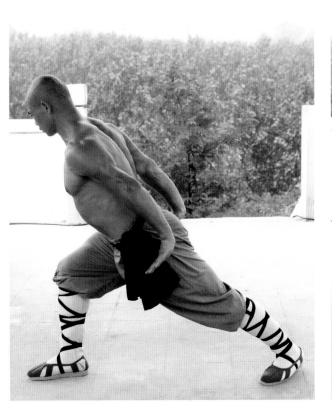 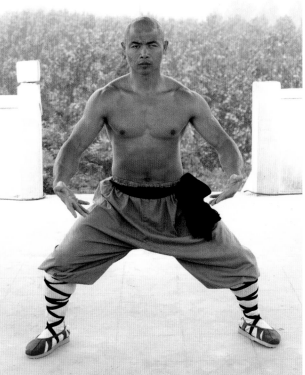

13) Go into Gong Bu. Push your palms down and push your head. Slightly tip your body over your right leg but make sure your back is straight.
REMAIN HERE FOR THREE BREATHS.

14) Inhale. Turn to the centre and go into Ma Bu.

YAO TOU SHI
TAKE YOUR SHOES OFF

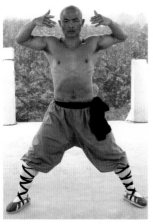 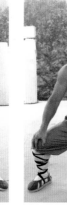 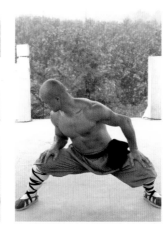 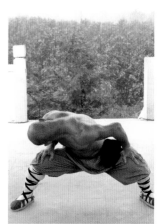

15) Come up a little higher and bring your hands to your head.

16) Exhale. Squat into Ma Bu and place your hands on both knees

17) – 19) Inhale. Drop your hips. Turn your upper body to the right. Leading with the neck, circle your body to the left.

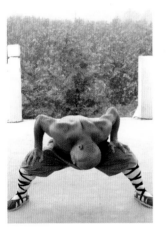

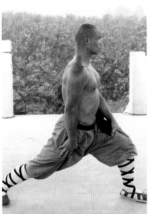

20) Exhale. Move into Gong Bu and raise your body. Left hand on your left knee, right hand inside your right leg.

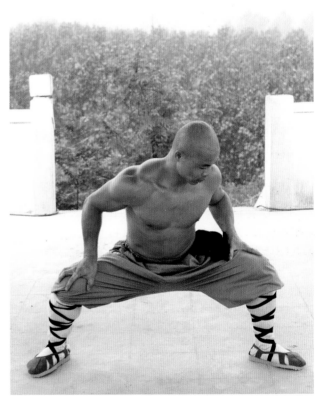

21) Inhale. Move into Ma Bu. Both hands holding your knee.

YAO TOU SHI
TAKE YOUR SHOES OFF

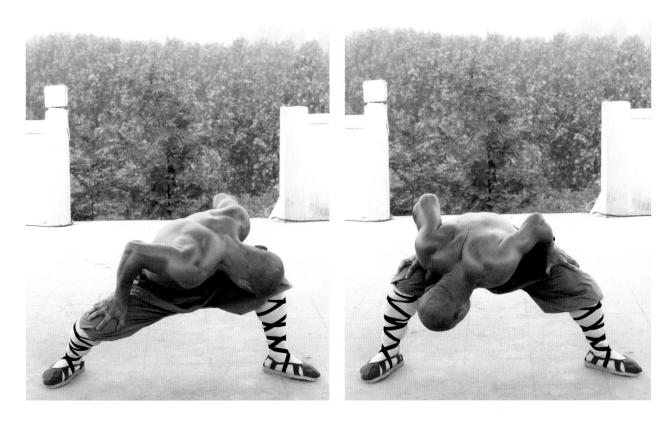

22) 23) Drop your hips. Leading with your neck, turn
from the left to the right.

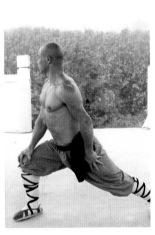

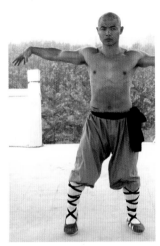

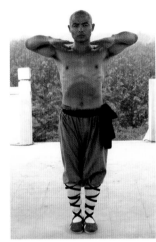

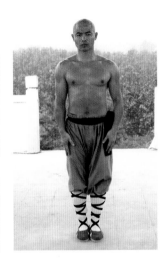

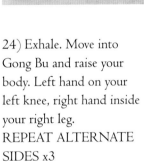

24) Exhale. Move into Gong Bu and raise your body. Left hand on your left knee, right hand inside your right leg.
REPEAT ALTERNATE SIDES x3

25) Inhale. Step your right foot in and raise your arms.

26) Close your feet and push your palms down.

27) Exhale. Stand straight. REMAIN HERE FOR THREE BREATHS.

5TH MOVEMENT

In this sequence you use your Qi to make your lower back go up into an arch. Sometimes this movement is called Lin Mao Gong Bei Shi – Cat Stretch Back. When you stretch your back, make sure that you curve upwards to activate a deep stretch in the back.

PAN JIAO SHI
HOLD YOUR FEET

START FROM NEUTRAL POSITION

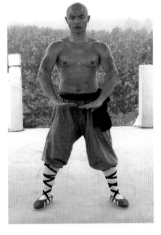 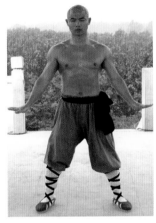 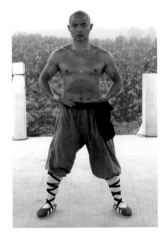 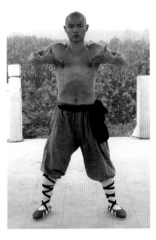

1) Step your left foot out to the side, at the same time bring your arms in front of your body and turn your hands so your palms face the ground.

2) Inhale. Keep turning your hands and bring them out to the side.

3) Continue to turn your hands and bring them to the front of your body, your palms facing the sky.

4) Draw your hands up your body.

PAN JIAO SHI
HOLD YOUR FEET

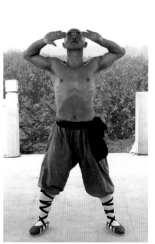 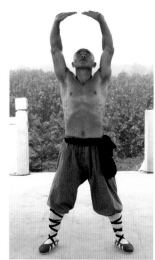 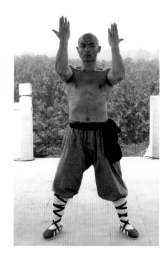 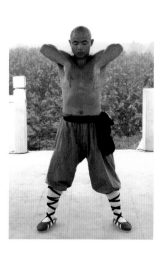

5) 6) Exhale. Push your palms up to the sky.

7) Inhale. Bring your palms down through the centre of your body.

8) Turn your palms so they face the ground and begin to exhale.

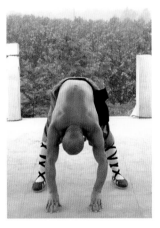 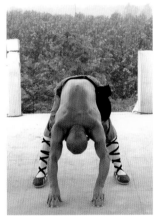 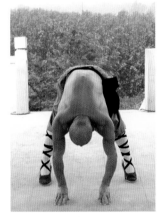 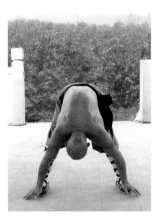

9) Fold forwards and touch the ground with your fingers, keeping your feet flat on the ground.

10) Inhale. Keep your fingers on the floor and your feet flat on the floor, and rock your body backwards.

11) Exhale. Push your fingers and rise up onto your toes, at the same time arch your back and allow your head to go into your body.

Use your stomach muscles to arch your lower back.

REPEAT STEPS 10 - 11 x3

12) Inhale. Hold your feet with your hands.

PAN JIAO SHI
HOLD YOUR FEET

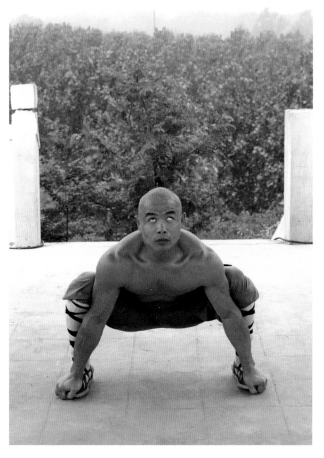

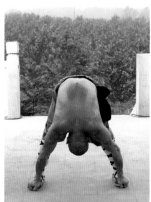

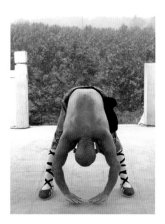

14) Exhale. Straighten your legs and arch your back. *Use your stomach muscles to arch your lower back.*

REPEAT STEPS 13-14
x3

15) 16) Inhale. Circle your palms by taking them out to the side and back to the centre.

13) Squat and lift your head up. Eyes look to the sky.

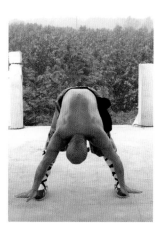 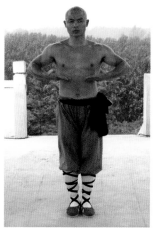 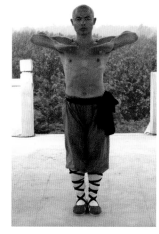 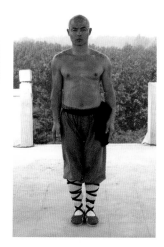

17) Come up slowly and bring your feet together. Palms facing the sky.
Make sure you come up slowly as if you come up too quickly you may get dizzy.

18) Exhale. Turn your palms to face the ground and push them down through the centre of your body.

19) Exhale. Stand straight. REMAIN HERE FOR THREE BREATHS.

6TH MOVEMENT

In this sequence you need to keep your eyes sharp and use internal and external energy. This is the only sequence when your eyes don't look peaceful. This movement helps you to gain energy. If you start to feel tired in Ma Bu you can raise the stance. When you have finished your punch and are turning the wrists, imagine that you are pulling something towards you.

ZHUAN QUAN SHI
CLENCH THE FIST

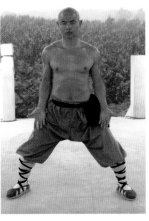
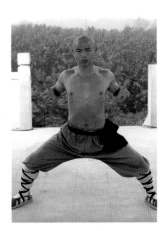
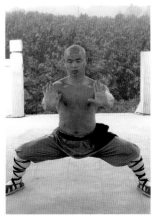
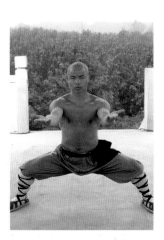

1) Inhale. Step your left foot out to the side and go into Ma Bu.

2) Squat down and draw your arms up.

3) Exhale. Turn your palms and push them straight out in front of you as hard as you can. This is low Ma Bu. *Make sure your feet grab the floor, your back is straight, your stance is stable.*

4) Inhale. Turn your palms to the sky.

ZHUAN QUAN SHI
CLENCH THE FIST

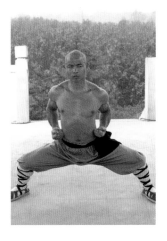 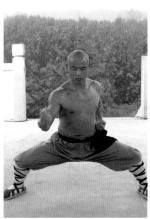 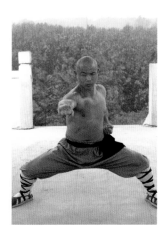 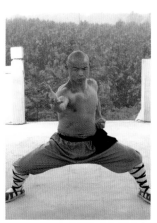

5) Bring your arms back to your waist. Make a fist with both hands.

6) Exhale. Slowly punch your right hand straight out in front of you.

7) When your arm is nearly straight, turn your wrist.

8) Inhale. Turn your hand and at the same time open your palm as if you are grabbing hold of something.

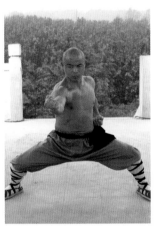 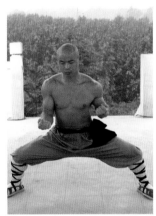 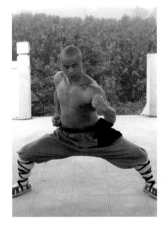 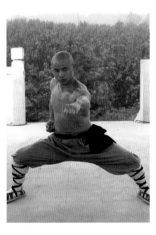

9) 10) Make a fist and pull it back to your waist.

Imagine you have a handful of small beans and you are trying to crush them.

11) Exhale. Slowly punch your left hand straight out in front of you.

12) Inhale. Turn your hand and at the same time open your palm as if you are grabbing hold of something. Turn your wrist, make a fist and pull it back to your waist. ALTERNATING FROM LEFT TO RIGHT, REPEAT THIS PUNCHING MOVEMENT x6 IN TOTAL.

ZHUAN QUAN SHI
CLENCH THE FIST

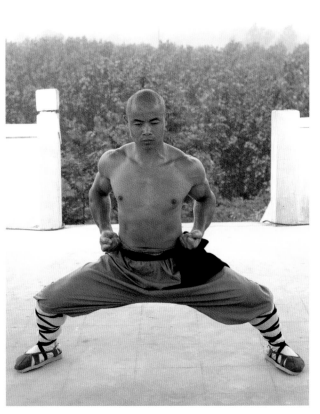

13) Inhale. Both fists at your waist.

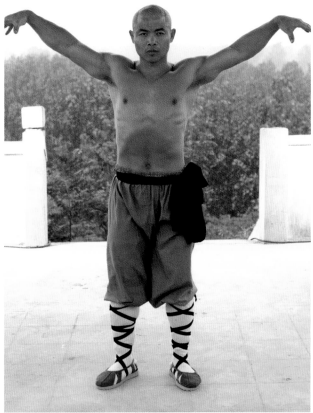

14) Step your left foot in and raise your arms.

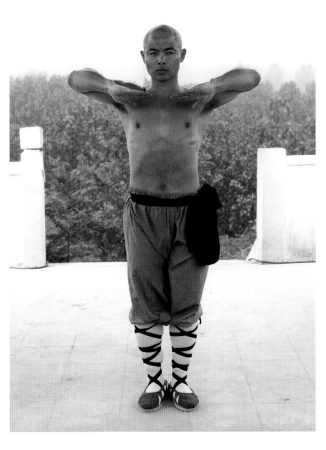

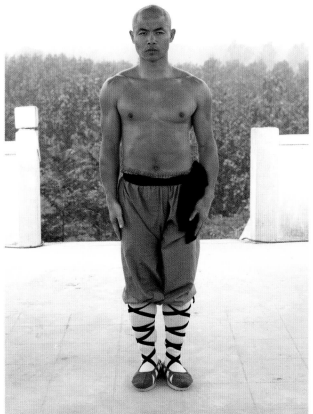

15) Push your palms down through your body and start to exhale.

16) Exhale. Stand straight.
REMAIN HERE FOR THREE BREATHS.

7TH MOVEMENT

In this sequence you need to use your heel to stamp and keep the rest of your body totally relaxed. At the same time as you stamp you need to push your palm downwards. When you stamp visualise that you are expelling all the toxins out of your body.

QI DIAN SHI
SEVEN STAMPS

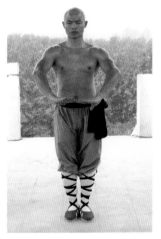 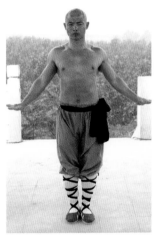 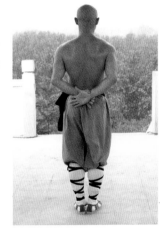 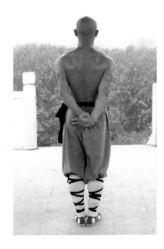

1) Inhale. Bring your arms in front of you, palms facing the ground.

2) Take your arms out to the side.

3) Clasp your left hand round the wrist of your right hand.

4) Exhale. Bring your shoulders back, keeping your back straight. Use your left hand to push your right hand down. *Make sure your back is straight and at the same time your head is pushing up.*

QI DIAN SHI
SEVEN STAMPS

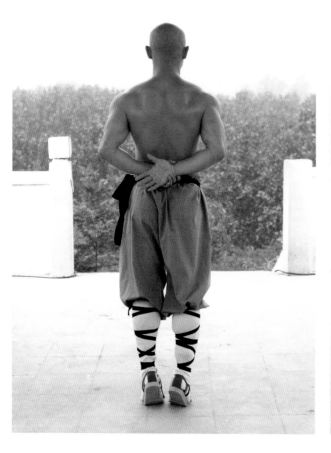

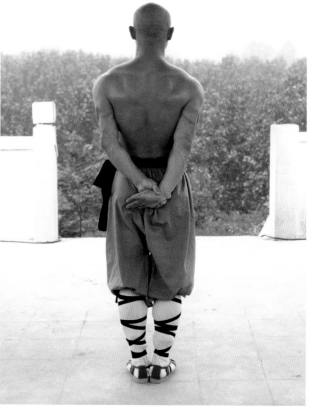

5) Rise up onto your toes. Lift your hands to your kidneys.

6) Exhale. Stamp down onto the heels of your feet and at the same time push your hands down.
REPEAT STEPS 5-6 x3

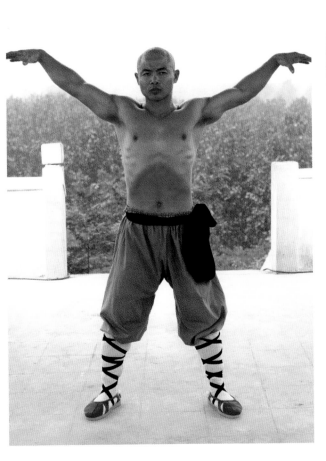

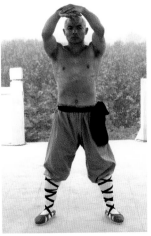

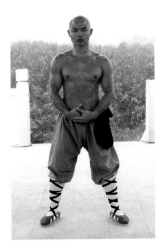

8) Clasp your hands together and bring them over your body – left hand on top of your right hand.

9) Exhale. Bring your arms down onto your stomach.

7) Inhale. Step your left foot out to the side. Bring your arms out to the side and raise your arms until they are over your head.

QI DIAN SHI
SEVEN STAMPS

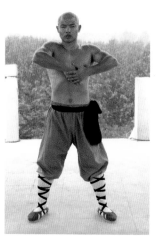 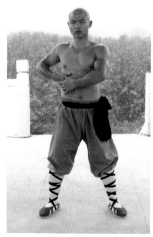 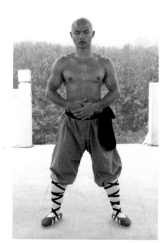 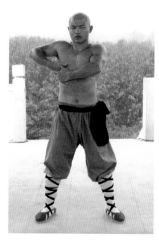

10) – 12) Inhale. Make a slow circle over your stomach in a clockwise direction, inhaling for the first half of the circle, as you go up and exhaling for the second half as you go down.
REPEAT x7

13) – 15) Change direction and make a slow circle in an anti-clockwise position.
REPEAT x7

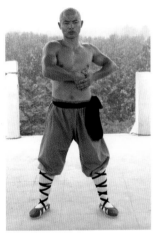 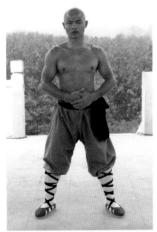 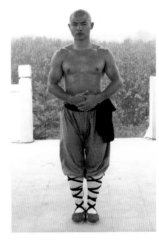 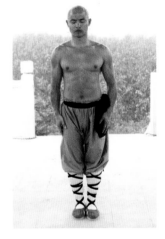

16) Step your left foot to your right foot.

17) Drop your arms. Stand straight. Close your eyes. Exhale.
REMAIN HERE FOR THREE BREATHS.

8TH MOVEMENT

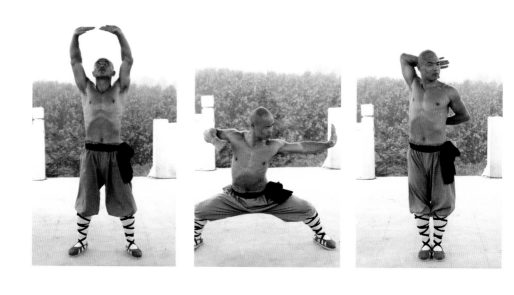

QUAN SHI
LINK TOGETHER

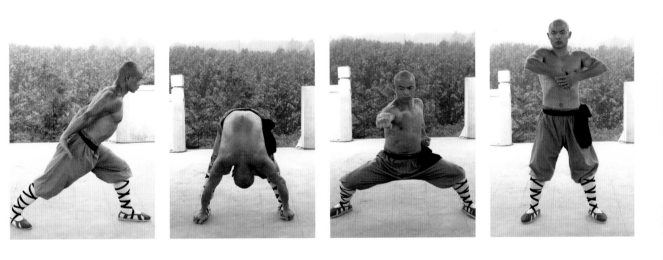

Once you know the movements, you then link up
sequence one through to seven. You can choose whether
to use three breaths in the neutral position. If your
breathing is strong and natural then you only need to
stand in neutral for one breath before continuing with
the next movement.

CHAPTER SIXTEEN

THE INSTANT HEALTH SELF-MASSAGE

It is beneficial to finish your practise with a self-massage as it greatly increases the power of Qigong. The 108 or 54 bamboo rods in the brush create vibrations which help to relieve stress and tension in the muscles, assist in unblocking the meridian channels, and help the body to detoxify through the stimulation of the lymphatic system.

The bamboo brush is for health and longevity. The metal brush is for martial artists and helps their body to become like stone on the inside and outside. At the Shaolin Temple, we say Qigong gives us a diamond body. Diamond body has two meanings; the first is for kung fu – this means we have good body conditioning so we can take punches and blows without getting injured. The other meaning is that our body and mind are peaceful, nothing can disturb us and disease cannot enter our body.

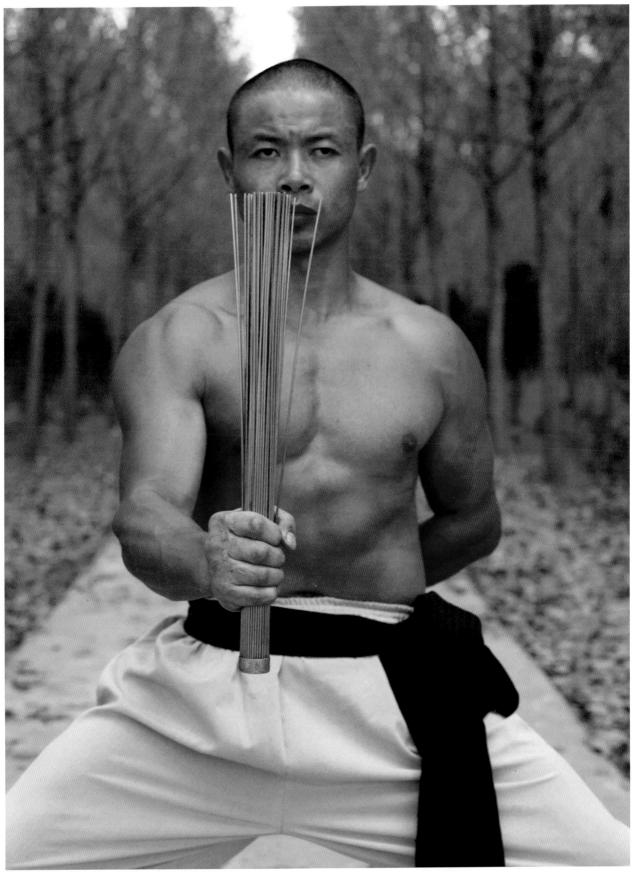

When you use the brush, you need to use your wrist rather than your arm. Try to use the top part of the brush not the middle. Repeat each section three times. The first time acts like a warm up and the second time you can use a little more power.

The first time we do it, we cleanse our skin but as we continue to do it more often and are able to use more power we move onto the final aim, which is to clean the bone. If bits of the bamboo break off then you are doing the massage correctly. This doesn't apply to the face and head, be gentle and make sure that you keep your eyes closed.

It is important that you cover every part of your body with the brush. If you look at the way the scales of a fish overlap each other, this is how we need to do the massage. You don't need to do this massage slowly but you can build up speed.

The massage usually takes about 10 – 15 minutes. That is all the time you need. There is no benefit from doing it for any longer than this.

It is best to wear light clothes or if you are in your own room you can wear your underwear and bare feet. You will find that this massage softens the skin. After doing the massage you will feel invigorated as if you have stepped out of a cold shower.

Practicing Qigong with this Instant Health Massage is the quickest way to get healthy, stay young and have a long life.

REMEMBER

When you massage with the brush there may be a feeling tenderness from some of the energy points but there should be no pain. Try to use your wrist when you beat yourself and keep an even rhythm, neither speeding up nor slowing down. Repeat three times on each part of your body.

CARE OF THE BRUSH

Do not share the brush with anyone else. Each practitioner needs to have his or her own brush. Because it's a natural product, it will wear down and need replacing. If you use it often then it's advisable to change it every six months. Keep it in a clean dry place away from dust. For safety reasons keep the brush away from children. You can purchase this brush from my website, details at the back of the book.

THE INSTANT
HEALTH MASSAGE

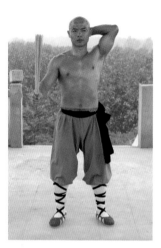 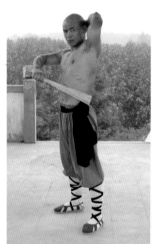 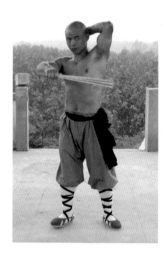

1) Open your feet a little and raise your right hand to your head to open the left side of your ribs.

2) 3) Moving in an upwards direction massage your ribs from the bottom to the top.

4) Change sides and repeat.

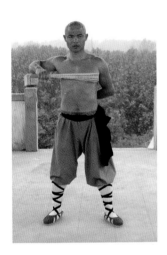 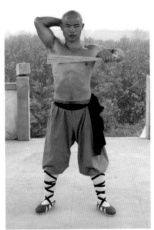

5) Massage in an upward direction from your stomach to your chest.

6) Change sides and repeat.

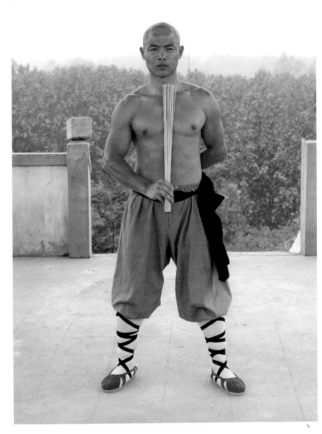

7) Massage along the middle of your chest.

THE INSTANT
HEALTH MASSAGE

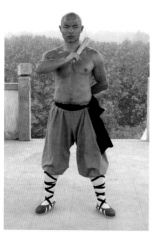 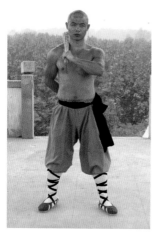 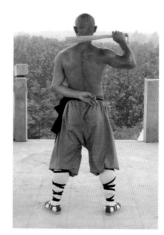 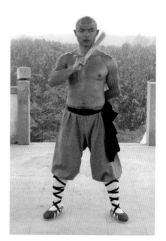

8) Massage both shoulders.

9) – 12) Circle the brush around your neck.

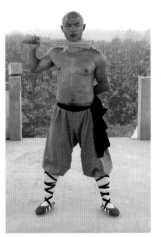 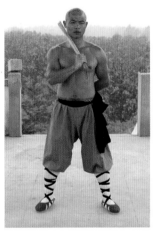 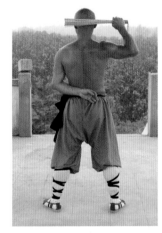 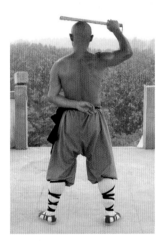

13) – 15) Massage your head from your lower head to the top of your forehead.

THE INSTANT
HEALTH MASSAGE

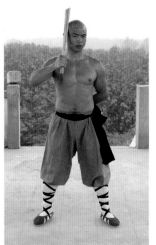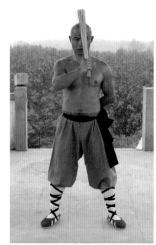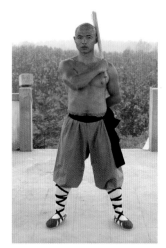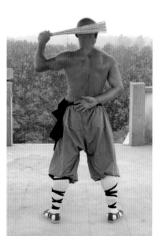

16) – 19) Circle the brush around the top of your head.

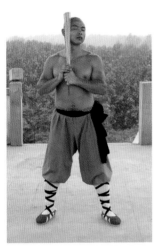 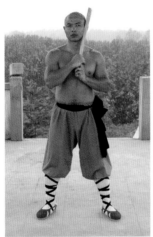 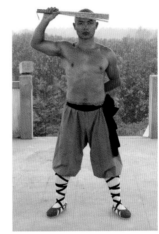 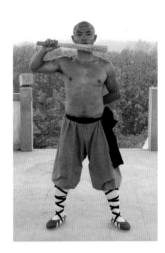

20) – 23) Massage your
face on each side and from
the forehead to your chin.

THE INSTANT
HEALTH MASSAGE

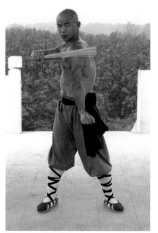 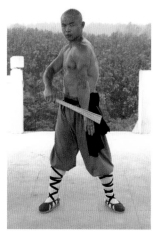 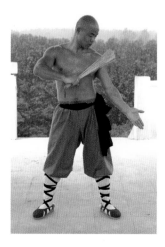 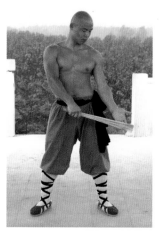

24) 25) Slightly turn your arm and massage the side of your arm all the way down to the tops of your fingers.

26) 27) Turn your arm and massage the inside of your arm and along the palm to the tips of your fingers.

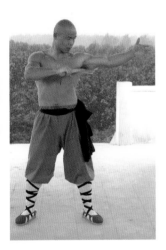 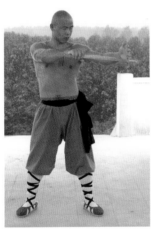 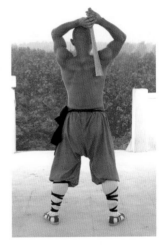 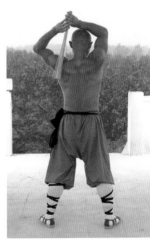

28) 29) Lift your arm and massage from your armpit and along the outside of your hand to your little fingers.
Repeat 24 – 29 on your other arm.

30) 31) Massage your upper back.

THE INSTANT
HEALTH MASSAGE

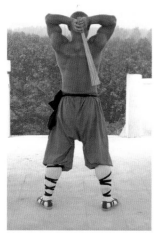 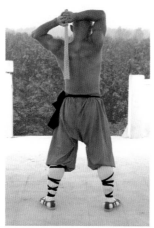 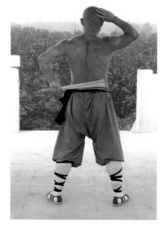 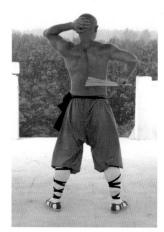

32) 33) Massage the
middle of your back.

34) 35) Massage your
lower back including your
kidneys.

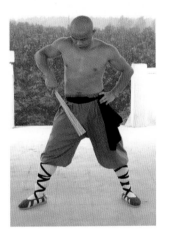 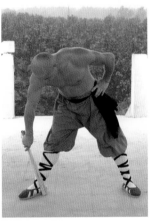 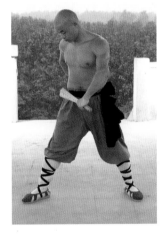 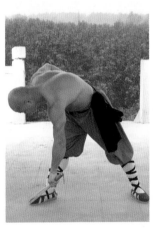

36) 37) Widen your legs a little and massage the inside of your leg all the way down to your big toe.

38) 39) Massage the front of your leg and across the top of your feet.

THE INSTANT
HEALTH MASSAGE

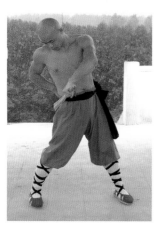 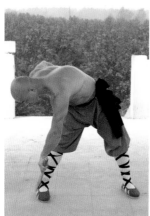

40) 41) Massage your outer leg all the way down to your little toe.

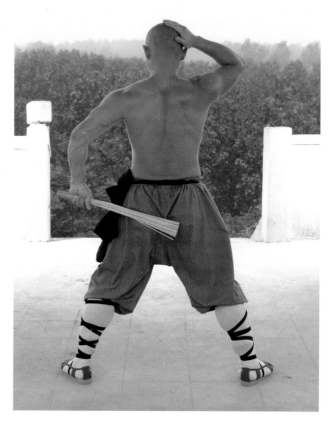

42) 43) Massage from your bottom and all the way down the back of your leg to your heel.
REPEAT 36 – 43 ON THE OTHER LEG.

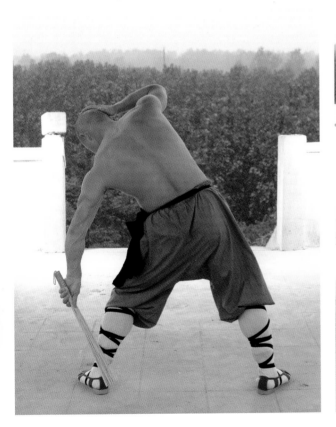
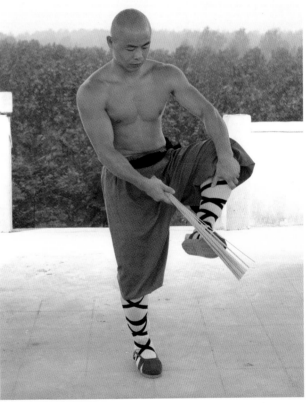

44) Massage the soles of both feet.

CHAPTER SEVENTEEN

HOW TO CONTINUE YOUR SHAOLIN QIGONG WORKOUT

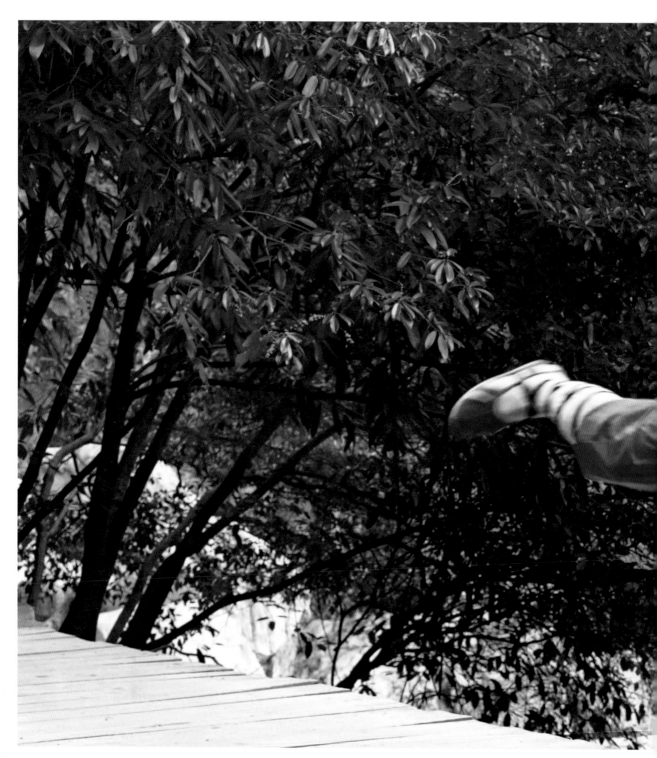

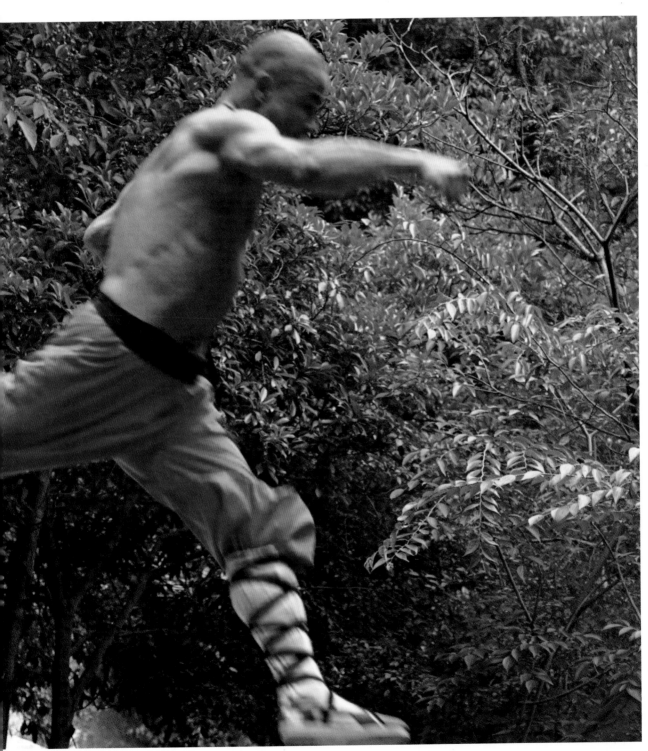

Whatever your goal, whether it is to become enlightened, be a millionaire, give something back to the world or be a great parent. The only way to achieve this is through having good health and optimal energy.

The exercises in this book give you the key to achieving this. Each time you workout you are unlocking the health and energy that is already within you. You don't need to go to a mountain or a temple to practise, you just need to practise right here and now. The place is not important, what is important is where your heart-mind is.

There will be days when it is easier to workout than others. This is natural. Life is about change and growth, and your practise will reflect this. When your mind is clogged up with stress and worry, remind yourself that each of us is a Universe and it's only when we empty ourselves of our mental chatter that we can then connect with the boundless Universal Energy. Let your Instant Health Workout be your refuge.

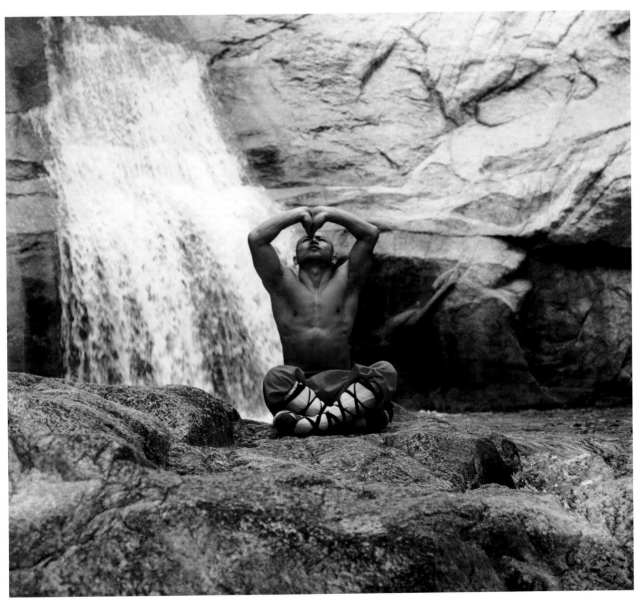

Just as Buddhists dedicate their meditation practise to benefit all beings in the world, you too can dedicate your practise to someone who is ill or going through a hard time. This act of dedication shifts the focus from the small "I" to the universal. In this way, your practise is not only a meditation but also a prayer.

My series of books are divided into two — Internal and External but really they are one. The practise of Qigong and the practise of Kung Fu is the same and for Instant Health you need to do both Qigong and Kung Fu (or some form of cardiovascular and strength training exercise). Make a strong plan and do what you can. When we do kung fu, if we can't do ten push-ups we start with five, and if we can't run ten miles we start with one. Qigong is the same; we step onto the path and slowly build up. The important thing is to start.

We know that our breath needs to be slow, even and deep but this won't happen straight away. We can only achieve this through patience and regular practise.
Let go of judgments in the practise, don't allow perfectionism or competitiveness to creep in, remember: You already are what you want to become.

Once you have learnt the whole of The Eight Treasures form, you can then begin to change the order of the sections around and make this form your own. If you have some imbalance in your body don't focus on these, and don't focus on where the Qi is going. Simply focus on the breath with the movement together. That's all you need to do. It's simple.

TRUST YOURSELF AND OVER TIME YOUR BODY WILL BECOME ITS OWN DOCTOR.

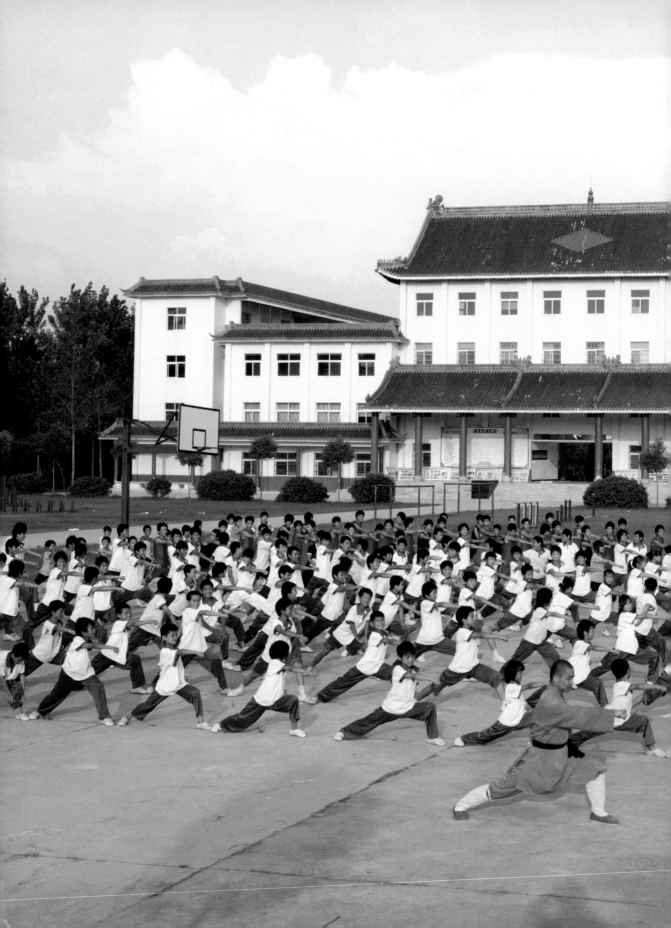

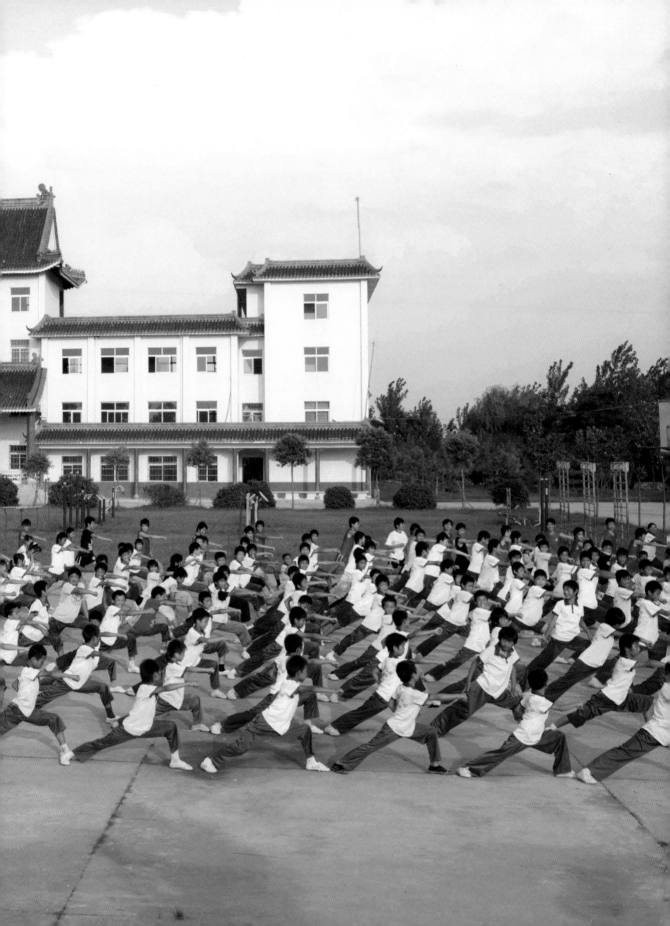

References

Mintel Healthy Lifestyle Report 2008
Scientific Reports
www.pubmed.gov
www.qigoninstitute.org

Yan Lei Press and Productions are dedicated to making available authentic teachings from the Shaolin Temple in China. We publish our titles and DVDs with the understanding of the Shaolin Arts as a living philosophy which is for the benefit of not only martial artists but all beings. For more information or to purchase any of our titles or equipment including The Instant Health Shaolin Massage Brush please visit:

WWW.SHIFUYANLEI.CO.UK

YAN LEI